THE ULTIMATE GUIDE TO TEACHER WELL-BEING

THE ULTIMATE GUIDE TO TEACHER WELL-BEING

BY

BENJAMIN DREER-GÖTHE
University of Erfurt, Germany

Foreword by John Hattie

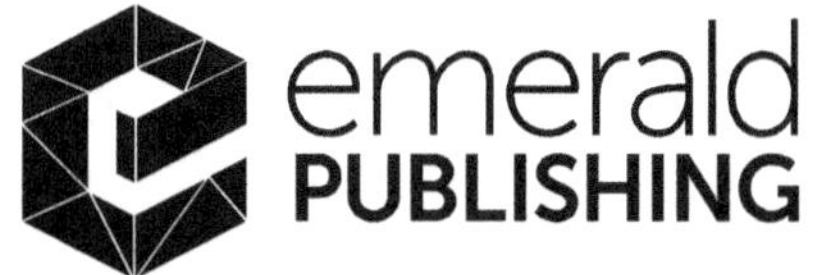

United Kingdom – North America – Japan – India
Malaysia – China

Emerald Publishing Limited
Emerald Publishing, Floor 5, Northspring, 21-23 Wellington Street, Leeds LS1 4DL.

British Library Cataloguing in Publication Data
A catalogue record for this book is available from the British Library

ISBN: 978-1-83742-060-5 (Print)
ISBN: 978-1-83742-057-5 (Online)
ISBN: 978-1-83742-059-9 (Epub)

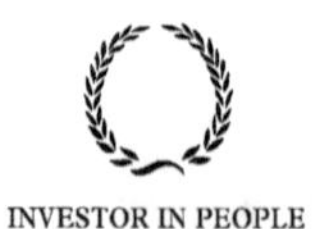

This book is dedicated to my wife – the finest teacher I know, both in the classroom and in life.

CONTENTS

FOREWORD BY JOHN HATTIE

I have three conundrums to introduce this book.

First, it seems that every week brings a new headline about the 'crisis' in teacher well-being, workload, attrition, or stress. Headlines such as *'School principals reaching crisis point, pushed to the edge by mounting workloads, teacher shortages, and abuse'* and *'Top teachers urge better pay and flexibility to address staff shortages'* dominate public discourse. While these claims of burnout and stress are well documented, they have also become weapons – narratives that can make teaching appear increasingly unattractive as a profession. Moreover, by continually legitimizing and amplifying talk about stress and burnout, we risk intensifying their psychological impact on educators already feeling depleted.

The issues of teacher and school leader workload and burnout are hardly new. Evidence shows that educators' time on task has changed little over the past 50 years. Give a teacher a group of students, a curriculum, and clear learning goals, and there will never be enough time to achieve all the desired academic, social, and emotional outcomes. This is the nature of teaching. Some argue that teachers are *time poor* – an unhelpful claim, since we all have the same amount of time. A more accurate description, as noted by Greene (1984), is that teachers *work in the present.* Their personal, social, emotional, and intellectual energies are fully focused *in the moment* – on creating the best possible conditions for learning. Any additional demands, no matter how well intentioned, can fragment that focus, create stress, and pull attention away from their core purpose: teaching. In this sense, teachers are easily overloaded and have good reason to feel that workload pressures are real and persistent.

What happened during and after the COVID-19 pandemic intensified the sense of angst, stimulated new conversations about social and emotional learning, and renewed attention to teacher well-being. My hypothesis is that the experience of teaching from home taught educators that teaching did not have to be so relentless. Working online allowed them brief moments of balance – time for a coffee, to put on a load of washing, or to play with the dog. They learned to teach students to work independently or collaboratively without their constant hovering and oversight. Breaks became genuine pauses rather than more conversations about school issues. But when lockdowns ended and teachers returned to classrooms, the old intensity returned with full force. Unlike many professions, teaching reverted to its traditional relentlessness. Teachers are now saying, in effect, 'enough'. The problem is not simply workload – it is *relentlessness*.

Second, more than 40 years ago, Lazarus and Folkman (1984) and others demonstrated that it is not the stressors themselves that determine outcomes, but the coping strategies individuals use in response to the stressors. The same stressor can elicit very different reactions depending on how it is appraised and managed. In the context of teacher well-being, the key issue is therefore not the presence of stress – an inevitable part of school life – but the nature and quality of the coping strategies teachers employ to deal with it. This is not about shifting blame to teachers; rather, it is an acknowledgement of the remarkable coping capacities educators demonstrate, often exceeding those found in many other professions.

Third, several meta-analyses have examined the relationship between teacher well-being and student achievement. For example, Maricuţoiu et al. (2023), drawing on 26 studies, reported a modest average correlation of $r = 0.07$ between the two. This small effect should not be interpreted as evidence that teacher well-being is unimportant. On the contrary, it suggests that teachers, as professionals, are remarkably capable of compartmentalizing their personal well-being to maintain effective classroom performance. The implication is that improving teacher well-being is unlikely to result from simply changing classroom behaviours or instructional techniques. Instead, it requires identifying and addressing the specific well-being challenges teachers face at a personal and systemic level.

Teaching has always been a profession defined by paradox: deeply rewarding yet profoundly demanding. In this book, *The Ultimate Guide to Teacher Well-Being*, Benjamin Dreer-Göthe bridges these tensions with rare clarity, offering a comprehensive, research-grounded, and profoundly human exploration of what it means for teachers to thrive.

This book is born from a decade-long inquiry into a deceptively simple question: *What can we actually do to support teacher well-being?* Dreer-Göthe shows that the answer lies not in slogans or self-care mantras, but in a multilevel system that joins policy, school culture, and individual practice. He dismantles three pervasive myths – the *martyr myth* (that teaching is noble suffering), the *peace of mind myth* (that well-being is calm detachment), and the *self-care myth* (that well-being is a personal task detached from context) – and replaces them with a richer, collective understanding.

Built around the Job Demands–Resources Model, Seligman's PERMA framework, and Ryff's model of psychological well-being, the book moves systematically across three interconnected levels: **policy**, how systemic levers such as workload regulation, pay, class size, and teacher voice shape the conditions of work; **school leadership**, how culture, collegial trust, appreciation, and shared meaning form the daily climate in which well-being lives or dies; and **individual teachers**, how self-acceptance, autonomy, emotional intelligence, and purpose foster resilience and growth.

Each of the 39 evidence-based measures is presented with a *Measure Dashboard* summarizing impact, quality of evidence, context dependency, sustainability, and feasibility, and each is illustrated through 55 real-world good-practice examples from 27 countries. The structure allows readers to navigate vertically (by system level) or horizontally (by theme), making the book equally valuable to policymakers, school leaders, researchers, and classroom practitioners.

What distinguishes this guide is its refusal to reduce well-being to comfort or to individual effort. It recognizes that teachers do not thrive *despite* challenges but *through* them – when those challenges occur in environments of trust, respect, and shared purpose. Thus, it is the coping strategies that need the focus. Teacher well-being is both a moral imperative and a strategic necessity – essential for student learning, school improvement, and the long-term vitality of education systems.

Ultimately, *The Ultimate Guide to Teacher Well-Being* is more than a handbook; it is an invitation – to rethink what we value in teaching, to design systems that honour the people who sustain them, and to act on the conviction that when teachers flourish, everyone benefits.

My three conundrums – the crisis narrative that fuels relentlessness, the recognition that coping strategies matter more than stressors, and the finding that teacher well-being exerts only a modest direct effect on student achievement and therefore must be treated sui generis as an important issue for the teachers – together illuminate the central challenge that *The Ultimate Guide to Teacher Well-Being* addresses. Dreer-Göthe shows that the future of teaching depends not on eliminating stress or chasing balance, but on reshaping the systems and cultures that determine how teachers experience and respond to their work. His analysis restores agency to educators, placing coping not as endurance but as professional artistry supported by thoughtful policy, empowering leadership, and humane working conditions. In doing so, the book reframes well-being as a collective achievement – one sustained when teachers are trusted, valued, and enabled to thrive in the midst of the inevitable demands of their vocation.

John Hattie, Melbourne Laureate Professor Emeritus

PREFACE

This book has both a short and a long history. The long history involves one of the most formative professional experiences I've had. About 10 years ago, I faced a decision about how to fulfil my university teaching obligation. I chose to offer a seminar on workload and stress for future teachers. My goal was twofold: to inform prospective teachers about the demands of their future profession and, in a collaborative effort, to explore and co-create new working time models that would better suit the needs of the next generation of educators. I spent countless hours preparing the new course and reviewing studies on burnout, stress models, and examples for inspiring alternative working time models. That course, however, was a failure. My students were neither ready to confront the challenges that lay ahead nor interested in questioning or redesigning the established structure of teachers' working hours. Most of them had accepted the current model as a given when they chose to become teachers. In addition, they weren't preoccupied with potential stress or strain. Instead, they were fuelled by optimism, driven by a sense of purpose, and focused on what they could accomplish in their future roles.

This disconnect forced me to reconsider my approach. If I wanted to support future teachers, I had to view their professional lives more holistically. It wasn't enough to highlight stressors like high noise levels or difficult student behaviour, although research has repeatedly shown these to be the most demanding issues for beginning teachers. I had to acknowledge the other side as well: the joy of seeing students learn, the satisfaction of contributing to someone's growth, the pride of being recognized as part of the school community. Hence, the focus on the positive was a better start, after all. Ultimately, this shift in perspective led me to the topic of teacher well-being. The more I explored it, the more I felt that this concept gave language and legitimacy to the complex reality of teaching. Teacher well-being, as I came to understand it, doesn't frame the positive and negative aspects of the profession as opposing forces. Instead, it embraces the idea that struggle, effort, joy, and pride are all integral parts of the teaching experience. Teachers don't thrive despite the challenges; they thrive through them. They invest in human relationships, take emotional risks, offer trust to students who may not yet know how to return it. That realization was an eye-opener for me, and I immediately knew then that teacher well-being would become my long-term research passion. Years later, in conversations with teachers, educators, and policymakers, I'm often asked the same question: 'Benjamin, what can we actually do to support teacher well-being?' Despite having conducted numerous studies and reviewed much of the literature, I still find this a difficult question to answer in a definitive, research-informed way. There is no universally agreed-upon 'menu' of measures, no equivalent to Hattie's Visible Learning that ranks the most effective strategies for enhancing teacher well-being. More and more, I started wondering why this is actually the case.

The answer, I have come to believe, is complex. It is not that there is a lack of research, nor is it due to a lack of interest or urgency. On the 'have' side, we already possess a substantial and growing body of literature on teacher well-being. Internationally, there are numerous publications, frameworks, and reflective accounts that recognize the importance of the topic. Many teachers, researchers, and other education professionals are actively contributing to this conversation. Their efforts indicate that the need for guidance and support is widely felt and sincerely addressed. However, on the 'missing' side, we lack clarity about what exactly we mean when we talk about teacher well-being. This conceptual vagueness is evident in both academic research and public discourse. In research, definitions of teacher well-being vary widely across studies, sometimes being treated as emotional satisfaction, sometimes as psychological resilience, sometimes as job satisfaction or work–life balance. These varying interpretations make it difficult for researchers to build a coherent body of knowledge or develop cumulative insights across studies. They also impede public discourse, where the term 'teacher well-being' is frequently invoked but seldom carefully defined or unpacked. It is often used rhetorically as something we ought to care about, but without much specificity. It risks becoming a catch-all term that can be used to justify anything from mental health workshops to staff appreciation days. After thinking about this for a while, it dawned on me that if there were to be a serious, research-informed guide on how to support teacher well-being, it would have to offer a way through this conceptual ambiguity first.

The short history of this book begins at a conference where I was struck by a comment that has stayed with me. During a presentation on teacher well-being, an Australian colleague remarked that many teachers in their system were experiencing what she called 'well-being fatigue'. She explained that teachers had grown weary of the constant emphasis on self-care and personal resilience. While they were being encouraged to attend workshops on mindfulness or to practise meditation after hours, the broader policy environment continued to allow actual working conditions in schools to deteriorate. That comment hit a nerve. It captured a growing disconnect I had also sensed in conversations elsewhere: the feeling that well-being has been reduced to an individual responsibility, while the structural and cultural factors that shape teachers' daily realities remain unaddressed. Again, if this were to be a serious, research-informed guide on how to support teacher well-being, it would have to go far beyond targeting teachers alone. It would need to be grounded in a multilevel perspective that recognizes that teacher well-being is neither created (nor diminished) in isolation.

In your hands, you now hold the result of this journey, somehow 10 years in the making, yet with a clear focus. This book is my attempt to bring together what research has taught us about teacher well-being while also clearing up the conceptual fog that so often clouds the discussion. The book does not focus solely on teachers, nor does it reduce well-being to individual self-care routines. Instead, it aims to weave together the multiple layers that shape what it means for teachers to thrive in their profession. That being said, this book is not meant to be a quick-fix manual. It is not a collection of 'tips and tricks' to help teachers feel better on a Friday afternoon. Rather, it is an invitation to reflect, to understand, and to act with greater clarity. I hope it will serve equally as a resource for teachers, school leaders, policymakers, and researchers who want to think more deeply and work more intentionally on creating environments where teacher well-being can flourish.

ACKNOWLEDGEMENTS

I wish to express my deep gratitude to Professor Sandra Neumann and the team of the Erfurt School of Education, whose generous support and consideration made it possible for me to devote the necessary time and care to this project. I am also grateful to Pam Firth for her exceptional editorial work on this manuscript.

This book is supported by Open Access funds of the University of Erfurt.

1

INTRODUCTION

In 1924, the management of the Hawthorne Works plant of the Western Electric Company in Cicero, Illinois, initiated a series of experiments. The aim was to explore whether worker productivity could be improved by adjusting the conditions in the factory. Harvard researcher Elton Mayo was appointed to oversee the investigations. In one of the early experiments, workers were divided into two groups; in one group, the lighting was gradually reduced over time, and in the other, the lighting remained constant. The group working under diminishing light conditions began to complain when it became nearly impossible to see. Surprisingly, until then, both groups showed a slow but steady increase in productivity in inspecting parts, assembling relays, and winding coils. The researchers concluded that lighting, as long as it met a minimal threshold, had no substantial impact on performance. Something else was influencing the workers' output.

Further experiments followed. In one, the researchers varied work and rest schedules and again measured productivity. The result? Another steady increase in performance, regardless of the schedule. The search for relevant causes continued. What ultimately stood out were the informal comments recorded from the workers. These suggested a powerful explanation for the observed increases in productivity: the improved social atmosphere and relationships among coworkers. Based on their observations, Roethlisberger and Dickson (1939) concluded that rather than environmental tweaks, social dynamics were driving performance gains. This marked a significant shift in how the conditions of work were understood. Later analyses expanded the initial explanation, pointing not only to the social fabric of the workplace but also to factors like the attention from researchers, the perceived privilege of participating in an experiment, and the increased communication with supervisors (Wickström & Bendix, 2000).

The phenomenon where productivity rises in response to being treated with special regard became known as the Hawthorne Effect (J. R. P. French, 1953), one of the most frequently cited findings in organizational psychology. What the Hawthorne Effect revealed was something surprisingly human; when people feel seen, valued, and part of something meaningful, they tend to work better. This insight served as a foundational starting point for the Human Relations Movement, which emphasized the psychological and emotional needs of employees, the significance of interpersonal relationships, and the influence of informal group dynamics on workplace performance. Over time, the Hawthorne studies have been criticized for their methodological limitations and overinterpretation. Later, researchers Wickström and Bendix (2000) recognized that a variety of factors likely contributed to the observed productivity increases, including

- relief from harsh supervision,
- receiving positive attention,
- learning new ways of interacting,
- opportunities to influence work procedures,
- rest breaks,
- higher income, and
- reduced fear of job loss.

Significantly, these aspects of the quality of a person's experience in their work are what we now associate with occupational well-being, a concept that has since evolved from a fringe concern to a central issue in work and organizational research. In today's competitive landscape where organizations compete for the brightest minds and most dedicated workers, well-being has become more than a byproduct of good management. It has become a strategic value and a relevant attraction factor (Schulte & Vainio, 2010).

1.1. THE TURN TOWARDS TEACHER WELL-BEING

A century later, a strikingly similar dynamic unfolded, this time not in a factory but in educational systems during the COVID-19 pandemic. As classrooms moved online, the dominant concerns were technical and procedural: how to maintain instruction through digital platforms, how to replicate learning conditions remotely, and how to keep educational routines intact (Dreer & Kracke, 2021). Much like in the early Hawthorne experiments, it was generally assumed that teaching effectiveness during lockdowns depended primarily on environmental variables like digital lesson formats, adequate devices, and platform choice. But once again, a more human truth emerged. Educators' motivation and performance were influenced less by formal conditions than by the quality of emotional and relational support. When these were stripped away, the well-being, professional identity, and purpose of many educators suffered (Wood & Quickfall, 2024). In the early stages, especially during the first lockdown, public appreciation for teachers surged. Parents, now witnessing the complexities of motivating students, gained a newfound respect for the patience, adaptability, and skill teaching requires. However, this wave of appreciation proved to be temporary. By the time the second lockdown phase began, sentiments had shifted. With some prior experience of remote learning, many parents began to develop specific expectations regarding the quality, structure, and outcomes of online education (L. E. Kim et al., 2024). In that sense, the COVID-19 pandemic-related lockdowns acted as a powerful magnifying glass. They exposed the central role teachers play in sustaining educational systems and their need to feel seen, valued, and part of something meaningful. In this regard, the pandemic inspired a modern-day Hawthorne moment for teachers by highlighting yet again that the invisible conditions of care, trust, collaboration, and recognition are essential.

Since these events, teacher well-being has gained significant traction in public discourse and policy circles. The groundwork for this attention was laid in the previous decade, as major international organizations increasingly positioned well-being as a strategic priority. The United Nations, for example, places 'Good Health and Well-Being' as the third of its 17 Sustainable Development Goals (United Nations, 2015), while the World Health Organization (WHO) views well-being as an essential component of global health. This broader focus has carried over into education as well. The Organisation for Economic Co-operation and Development (OECD) Learning Compass 2030 frames 'well-being for all' as an educational outcome and guiding principle for designing and evaluating learning environments (OECD, 2019).

Another critical driver of this growing focus has been the teacher shortages now affecting many countries. These shortages have intensified existing pressures due to higher workloads and diminished resources. They have pushed policymakers to reexamine what makes the teaching profession attractive and sustainable (UNESCO & International Task Force on Teachers for Education 2030, 2024). As a result, teacher well-being ranks higher on the priority list for practitioners and policymakers. One concrete example is the European Commission's establishment of an expert group on well-being in schools, aimed at supporting the Directorate-General for Education, Youth, Sport and Culture in crafting evidence-based policy for EU member states.

This renewed attention has also fuelled a growing body of empirical research looking more closely at conditions, outcomes, and interventions related to teacher well-being.

1.2. THE RIPPLE EFFECT OF TEACHER WELL-BEING

Research results increasingly demonstrate that teacher well-being has far-reaching consequences for classrooms, school culture, and student outcomes (Dreer, 2023a). In that sense, the impact of occupational well-being can be understood as a ripple effect with wide-ranging and lasting consequences. Like a stone dropped into still water, the effects of teacher well-being extend far beyond the point of origin, touching classrooms, schools, and entire education systems. Drawing from a wide array of empirical studies, these effects can be visualized as six expanding circles or 'ripples' (see Fig. 1), each representing a level of influence that flows outward from the teacher at the centre.

The first ripple is the teacher themselves, their personal and professional functioning, including beliefs about their professional efficacy, mental and physical health, and key indicators like absenteeism or intentions to leave the profession (e.g. O'Reilly, 2014). The second ripple reflects how this internal state shapes visible teaching behaviour: the way teachers communicate, the methods they use, how they manage the classroom, and how they respond to student needs (e.g. Buonomo et al., 2019; Burić & Frenzel, 2020; Moè et al., 2010). The third ripple concerns the quality of instruction that students experience. When teachers are well, they create more emotionally supportive, cognitively stimulating, and motivationally engaging learning environments (e.g. Collie et al., 2012; Fouché et al., 2017; Kunter et al., 2013). The fourth

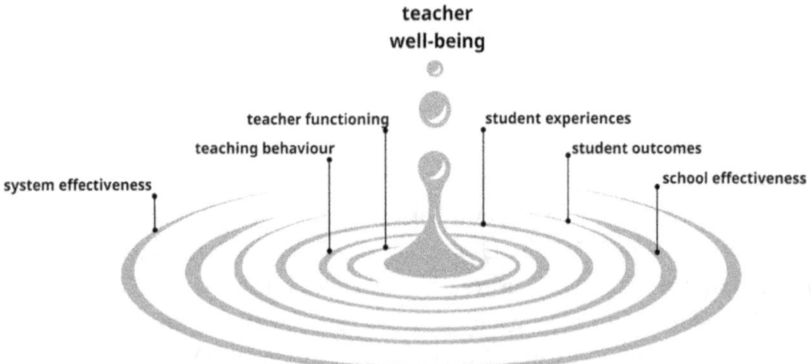

Fig. 1. Ripple Model of Teacher Well-Being. Figure Created by the Author.

ripple reaches student outcomes directly. This includes academic motivation and performance and how students generally feel and think about school (e.g. Caprara et al., 2006). The fifth ripple expands to the collective level: the shared well-being of teaching staff shapes school climate, supports professional collaboration, and fosters institutional trust and stability (e.g. Bajorek et al., 2014). Finally, the sixth and widest ripple touches the education system as a whole. Teacher well-being supports system resilience by reducing attrition, buffering teacher shortages, and fuelling improvement efforts. Taken together, these six ripples form a compelling model for understanding the depth and reach of teacher well-being. What begins as a personal experience becomes a professional condition, a pedagogical factor, a student outcome, a school culture, and a systemic force. Based on that visual, this book begins with a clear and important insight: Whether you care about the people behind the profession or focus on hard outcomes like student achievement and system performance, whether you're driven by ideals of educational efficiency or social justice, or whether you're a policymaker shaping reform or a grandparent hoping for a brighter future for your grandchildren – teacher well-being is something you should care about.

2

TEACHER WELL-BEING: A COLLECTIVE RESPONSIBILITY

Until now, the term *teacher well-being* has appeared several times in this book without a clear definition. This was intentional. In many cases, readers are quick to project their own ideas of well-being onto the text. And if the lack of a definition has not stood out so far, that may be exactly what has happened – you may have unconsciously filled in the blanks. The problem is that those blanks are often filled with common myths or oversimplified assumptions about what teacher well-being means. The easiest route would be to offer a broad definition and move on. But that is not the aim here. Doing so would simply offer another, albeit narrower, canvas onto which readers might project their existing misunderstandings. Without first challenging those misconceptions, even a well-crafted definition risks being misread or reduced to familiar, but inaccurate, ideas. Before going any further, it is worth pausing to examine those assumptions and to consider why subscribing to a single, fixed definition of teacher well-being may not be the best approach at all. With that in mind, let us now examine three persistent myths about teacher well-being and consider the implications they hold for the approach taken in this book.

2.1. THE MYTH OF MARTYR

A recent study asked more than 2,000 workers across the United States how they felt about their jobs. Most of them said they were quite satisfied. But when asked how they thought others were doing, their answers shifted. More than half believed that most other people were not satisfied at all (Glavin & Schieman, 2025). Does this sentiment resonate with you? That gap between how we feel and what we think others feel about work points to a longstanding belief many of us carry; work is meant to be hard, something we just must individually push through. Enjoying your job still feels like the exception. Even when people are content, they often assume they are one of the lucky few and that most others are just getting by. In this paradigm, work is often seen as a contest between the individual and the system, a confrontational relationship in which survival depends on one's capacity to harden oneself against the very conditions of the systems they work in. To succeed, one is expected to adapt to dysfunction, normalize stress, and cultivate resilience as a shield for withstanding it. The same narrative can be found for teachers:

> *It seems to be accepted as an article of faith that teaching is stressful, and commentators typically refer to the high numbers of people leaving the profession; and for those who remain in it, they chart the prevalence of chronic stress, anxiety, depression, poor physical health and even suicide ... Typically, discussion of 'teacher well-being' relates either to pay and conditions or to workplace health, and usually focuses palliatives to ease the stress of work or interventions to prevent illness and pathology. (Morris, 2015, p. 169)*

In the scientific literature, we find a dominant focus on the darker side of the teacher experience. For a long time, research tended to frame teacher well-being through the lens of stress, strain, and burnout (e.g. Cano et al., 2017; Collie et al., 2017; Travers, 2017). Even when interventions are proposed, they are often reactive in nature, centred on treating symptoms rather than addressing the underlying causes. Klusmann and Waschke (2018) expressed concern that nearly every publication on teacher well-being begins by justifying its importance through references to attrition, stress, or poor mental health, almost as if these problems are the only lens through which teacher well-being can be seen.

This framing has become particularly entrenched in the wake of the COVID-19 pandemic. As schools closed, workloads surged, and uncertainty reigned, researchers rushed to quantify the cost. Again, the questions focused on pressure and endurance: How much stress are teachers under? How close are they to burnout? These were necessary inquiries, and they generated important insights. But once more, the picture that emerged was narrow. Well-being became the absence of suffering rather than a state of vitality, connection, or professional joy. While it might be seen as a detail only geeky researchers obsess about, this 'myth of martyr' has important implications. It fuels the belief that improving teacher well-being primarily means reducing stress, strain, or burnout. As a result, efforts to support teachers will exclusively focus on stress reduction techniques, time management workshops, or mindfulness exercises. While such interventions may offer temporary relief, they fail to address the deeper, more holistic aspects of well-being. What this view overlooks is that true well-being is not just about minimizing harm. It is equally about creating the conditions in which teachers can flourish. This includes fostering positive emotions in the workplace, building meaningful relationships, cultivating a strong sense of purpose, and embedding a culture that celebrates growth and success. When well-being is understood in this fuller sense, the goal is not simply to help teachers cope but to enable them to thrive professionally, personally, and collectively.

Yet a quiet shift is underway. In recent years, researchers have begun asking more expansive and constructive questions. Between 2000 and 2019, the number of studies drawing on holistic frameworks increased significantly (Hascher & Waber, 2021). These frameworks conceptualize well-being as a multidimensional construct that encompasses not only the absence of stress and burnout, but also the presence of meaning, positive relationships, professional agency, and a sense of fulfilment. This represents a crucial turning point. More importantly, this shift provides a foundation for developing robust, evidence-based approaches to measuring teacher well-being in its full complexity, including both positive and negative dimensions. It also enables the design and evaluation of interventions that do more than reduce stress – namely, those aimed at actively cultivating positive conditions such as purpose, connection, and joy in teachers' professional lives.

2.2. THE PEACE OF MIND MYTH

If you search online for images related to well-being, alongside countless photos of people in meditative poses you will most likely also come across an illustration often used in mindfulness workshops (for example, here: https://www.coolmindshk.com/en/mindful-vs-mind-full/). It shows a person walking a dog through a calm landscape with four trees and the sun. Above them float two thought bubbles. The one on the left is crammed with symbols of tasks and worries ('mind full'), while the other simply reflects the peaceful landscape ('mindful'). The message seems clear: a calm mind equals well-being. Applied to teaching, this illustration would suggest that a teacher experiences well-being particularly when, in the midst of a chaotic and noisy classroom, they are able to retreat mentally into a peaceful inner space. This is understandable, since anyone working daily with restlessness, interruptions, and high expectations longs for complete serenity. Especially when one accepts that a permanently stress-free working day as a teacher is impossible, the idea becomes tempting that well-being can be achieved by meeting the inevitable hustle and bustle of the outside world with inner calm.

This perspective has severe consequences. First, it implies that teacher well-being should primarily be assessed according to how 'untouched' they appear by external challenges. The less they seem affected by their experiences at school, the more satisfied they should be with their professional situation. For interventions, a similar logic follows; measures aim to teach teachers to mentally block out external disturbances or to negate the experience of reality rather than to deal with challenges constructively. Teachers would therefore be encouraged to ignore the bustle of everyday life instead of shaping it productively. In practice, this myth can tempt teachers to withdraw from challenges, to avoid risks, and to shift responsibility for their professional lives, at least mentally, onto others.

The basic misunderstanding underlying the peace of mind myth is the assumption that teacher well-being primarily means mental tranquillity and serenity. Even the concept of mindfulness, which is often used as the basis for such assumptions, does not describe passive switching off but rather conscious presence in the current moment (Zarate et al., 2019). Interestingly, studies suggest that mindfulness practices can, in certain contexts, reduce the willingness to actively engage with new tasks or challenges (Hafenbrack & Vohs, 2018). When well-being is reduced solely to inner peace, the activating, energizing aspects of professional experience easily fade into the background. However, research findings clearly show that states such as enthusiasm, intrinsic motivation, or flow not only enhance professional performance but also contribute significantly to fulfilment and satisfaction (Olčar et al., 2019; Zilka et al., 2023).

In reality, well-being in the teaching profession is closely linked to engagement. Positive work experiences broaden cognitive and behavioural possibilities and contribute, in the long term, to building resources (Frenzel, 2014). These in turn foster or reinforce the motivation to take on new undertakings and projects (Fredrickson, 2001). Well-being is therefore characterized by vitality and by the intensive investment of mental and emotional energy in one's work (H. Yang et al., 2023). This includes, for example, the excitement of implementing new ideas and projects, the drive to question established norms, and the courage to explore innovative paths.

This scientifically informed understanding of well-being has clear implications. For one, vitality-related factors such as professional engagement should be considered indicators, while detachment – supposed inner calm – should be regarded as a detrimental facet. At the same time, externally imposed constraints become relevant; teachers may be highly motivated yet feel blocked by external conditions or caught up in tasks they consider meaningless. A comprehensive diagnosis of well-being should therefore not only capture the state of motivation but also include the perception of success and the achievement of professional goals. For interventions, the implication is that measures should primarily foster engagement and intrinsic motivation. For instance, this can be achieved through opportunities for autonomy, support for innovative projects, collegial networking, and constructive, appreciative feedback.

2.3. THE SELF-CARE MYTH

For the teaching profession, the image of the lone fighter has existed for a long time (Roeder, 1991). What happens behind closed classroom doors lies in the responsibility of the teacher. Only they can significantly shape the course of the lesson. Even during working phases outside of class, such as marking or preparing lessons at their desks at home, teachers are on their own. This image fits neatly with an already highly individualized guiding culture in Western societies, in which concepts such as self-determination, personal responsibility, and self-optimization are omnipresent (Acton & Glasgow, 2015). It is therefore unsurprising that people choose the teaching profession because they expect a high degree of autonomy in shaping their work (Eder et al., 2011). Ultimately, the ability to attribute success to oneself can be a decisive motivator in daily work (Ding & Rohlfs, 2020). In this context, it seems only logical that one's well-being, generally regarded as a personal matter anyway, should also fall within the teacher's individual responsibility. The thinking is: 'I take care of my lessons, my students, and certainly of my own well-being.' At first glance, seeing well-being as a purely personal task appears empowering – one simply needs to find the 'right' routines, attitudes, or tools to face the challenges of the profession and remain independent of the decisions or behaviours of others.

If we view well-being solely as the teacher's responsibility, this has direct consequences for diagnosis and intervention. In diagnostic terms, the focus then falls exclusively on subjective aspects, such as personal feelings in a given work situation or environment. Yet this provides hardly any information about the conditions influencing well-being, such as workload, class structure, support from colleagues, or the school's organizational framework. The timing of measurement also takes on disproportionate significance, since individual assessments can fluctuate and are additionally shaped by other areas of life (e.g. family circumstances). This, in turn, makes it easy for decision-makers to misinterpret impaired well-being as a passing mood that will resolve itself over time. If well-being is seen as solely the teacher's responsibility, interventions consequently focus only on individual coping strategies such as meditation, journaling, exercise, and practices of gratitude and kindness. These measures carry several problems: (1) Activities to improve well-being are not considered part of professional duties within this logic. They must therefore be organized, paid for, and undertaken in one's own time. (2) Each teacher decides individually whether to take part in support offers. As a result, those already well-informed often engage, while those in greatest need of support remain unreached. (3) Not every method suits every person, and finding the right techniques can be difficult. Prolonged searching or trying out multiple approaches may itself become an additional burden. (4) If, despite these practices, stress is not reduced or satisfaction not improved, feelings of personal failure may arise. (5) If teachers do not succeed in finding effective ways of managing challenges, specific strains may remain unaddressed and worsen over time. (6) The already existing pressure on teachers to constantly optimize their professional work (e.g. through ever better teaching methods) is further intensified by the notion that they must also fully manage their own well-being.

Considering the ripple effects of teacher well-being (see Introduction), which extend far beyond the health and performance of the individual teacher, there are compelling reasons for the school community, for education policy, and ultimately for society at large to take teachers' well-being seriously and to address it appropriately. This means it cannot be left solely to individual teachers to manage excessive professional stress single-handedly or to generate positive work experiences entirely on their own. Rather, structures, measures, and goals within schools and education systems must be aligned with the professional needs of teachers. A growing body of research shows that many of the challenges to teachers' well-being arise from systemic problems. These include, for example, excessive workload, rigid accountability requirements, lack of autonomy, insufficient leadership, and a poorly supportive social climate (McCallum, 2020; D. Price & McCallum, 2015). Such factors lie outside the control of individual teachers and cannot be remedied by personal effort alone.

The consequences of this understanding of shared responsibility for well-being are stark; both the individual experiences of teachers and the systemic conditions must be considered. For one, this means that alongside subjective perceptions such as stress and motivation, structural factors such as workload, autonomy, and support from colleagues and leaders must be incorporated into an overall picture of well-being. Moreover, interventions cannot target self-management alone; they must also include measures that improve working conditions, strengthen collegial support, and foster a culture in which well-being is systematically enabled. Importantly, teachers themselves do not always have to take an active role in driving these changes.

2.4. CONSEQUENCES FOR THIS BOOK

The previous chapter has demonstrated that there are compelling reasons for society to prioritize teacher well-being, but doing so requires a thoughtful and effective approach. To chart a better path forward, this book seeks to avoid the common misconceptions that have undermined past efforts. First, it adopts a holistic perspective on teacher well-being, one that recognizes the inherent demands while also embracing the energizing and meaningful aspects of the profession. Second, this book does not aim to make teaching effortless or stress free. Moreover, this book does not seek to provide teachers or school leaders with arguments for withdrawing from responsibility or shifting the blame onto higher authorities. Rather, it explores how to make this challenging work fair, engaging, meaningful, and fulfilling. It promotes an active, dynamic view of well-being that acknowledges adversity while finding value and growth in actively addressing it. Third, this book is not simply a guide for teachers on how to become more resilient in adverse conditions. It is written with equal attention to policymakers, school leaders, and teachers, recognizing that each plays a vital role in shaping the conditions under which teaching and learning thrive. To support this aim, the book outlines measures to enhance teacher well-being at three interrelated levels: policy, school leadership, and the individual teacher. These can be pictured as a set of matryoshka dolls, which are a set of wooden figures that fit inside one another (see Fig. 2). The largest doll represents policy, giving the set its outer contours, much like national and regional frameworks define the structural conditions of schooling. Inside sits the middle doll, held within that shape yet free to turn and shift. This reflects how school leaders and leadership teams interpret policy and shape the daily culture of their schools, with their agency and growth depending on the space and protective form provided by the outer doll. At the centre is the smallest figure, enclosed by the outer layers but still with space to move and turn. This represents the teacher whose professional agency and growth depend on the protective space and support provided by both the policy and leadership dolls.

While Fig. 2 depicts the dolls as a single set, a matryoshka can also be taken apart and each figure can be handled on its own. The following chapters

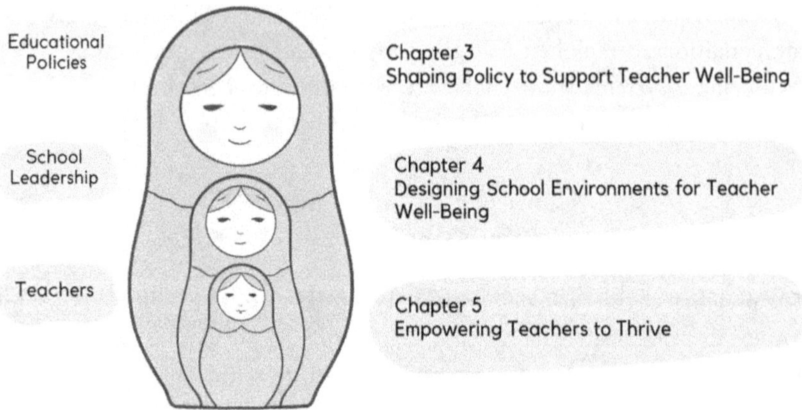

Fig. 2. Teacher Well-Being and Chapter Structure as a Matryoshka Doll System. Figure Created by the Author.

take this approach, and each level is unpacked and explored separately. Yet the analyses are always conducted with the complete set in mind, recognizing that teacher well-being is shaped by the space, support, and protective form provided by the surrounding dolls (levels). For examining each doll separately, the book embraces conceptual variety as a strength (Dreer-Goethe, 2025a). At each level, a distinct lens on teacher well-being is applied to ensure that the proposed measures align with the specific challenges and possibilities for change inherent to that part of the set.

Chapter 3 begins at the macro level, the outer shell. Although often invisible in the day-to-day routines of schools, policy decisions fundamentally shape the conditions under which teachers work and students learn. Based on the Job Demands–Resources (JD-R) Model by Demerouti et al. (2001), this chapter explores how job demands and resources are influenced by policy and examines what research reveals about designing policies that support, rather than strain, the teaching profession.

In Chapter 4, attention shifts to the school level (the middle doll), where teacher well-being is shaped by everyday practices and culture. The chapter examines how Seligman's (2011) five pillars of well-being – positive emotions, engagement, relationships, meaning, and accomplishment – contribute to the professional flourishing of teachers.

Chapter 5 focuses on the individual level (the centre doll), exploring how personal agency is shaped by and responds to broader system conditions. Using Ryff's (1989) model of psychological well-being as a foundation, the chapter outlines measures to support teacher well-being by cultivating self-acceptance, utilizing autonomy, improving environmental mastery, clarifying and connecting with purpose, and engaging in personal growth.

Each chapter follows a consistent structure, beginning with a contextual overview and a level-specific definition of teacher well-being. This is followed by a series of in-depth subchapters, each presenting one distinct, research-backed measure. To support practical application, every measure is accompanied by a Measure Dashboard, a tool that outlines key parameters such as projected impact, context sensitivity, and sustainability. This enables readers to make informed decisions based on their priorities, whether they seek measures with the greatest potential impact or those that are more readily implementable. Additionally, each measure is illustrated with at least one good-practice example, demonstrating its real-world feasibility and offering a practical starting point for similar initiatives. Importantly, this book is firmly grounded in research. All proposed measures and interventions are supported by robust evidence. At the same time, the book recognizes the boundaries of existing research and refrains from drawing conclusions in areas where evidence remains limited, emerging, or inconclusive.

The measures presented in this book can be read from beginning to end or explored selectively, depending on your area of interest and level of engagement. To better understand how each measure is structured and situated, I recommend reading the introductory section and conceptual definition at the start of each chapter. However, if you are short on time and simply wish to browse the catalogue of measures, you are welcome to do so. At the end of the book, you will find a complete list of all measures without additional details such as the Measure Dashboards or good-practice examples. This overview allows for a quick scan of the suggested measures, making it easier to identify those most relevant to your needs and to dive deeper into the ones you select.

3

SHAPING POLICY TO SUPPORT TEACHER WELL-BEING

Addressing teacher well-being at the policy level requires a systematic approach that acknowledges the intricate interplay between workplace demands and available supports. The JD-R model, developed by Demerouti et al. (2001), offers such a framework. It moves beyond individual-level explanations and instead situates well-being within the broader design of work environments. At its core, the JD-R model recognizes that every job involves a mix of demands and resources. Job demands are defined as 'physical, social, or organizational aspects of the job that require sustained physical, cognitive and/or emotional effort and are therefore associated with certain physiological and psychological costs' (Demerouti et al., 2001, p. 501). In teaching, these demands include the inherent challenges that are embedded in the nature of the profession itself. These inherent demands are part and parcel of what it means to be a teacher. For example, teaching is, by definition, emotionally labour-intensive work (Molyneux, 2021). It requires constant interpersonal engagement, often with diverse groups of students, each with distinct learning needs, emotional states, and social backgrounds. This includes managing classroom dynamics, responding to student issues, and maintaining professional composure even in moments of disruption, resistance, or crisis (Tsouloupas et al., 2010). Cognitively, teaching requires a high level of adaptive expertise. Teachers must process and respond to complex information in real time, make countless instructional decisions over the course of a single day, and continuously adjust their approach to match the needs of individual students and whole-class dynamics. These are not routine or mechanical tasks; they require sustained concentration, deep pedagogical knowledge, and the ability to synthesize feedback on the fly. Moreover, the moral dimension of teaching adds a further layer of complexity. Teachers are often driven by a strong sense of purpose and responsibility. This moral imperative can heighten the emotional toll of the job, especially in contexts of inequality, trauma, or underresourcing. The weight of caring for, mentoring, and supporting students through their academic and personal growth is deeply meaningful but also inherently demanding.

By distinguishing between such inherent demands that are intrinsic to the role and those that are structural and modifiable (such as excessive workload or bureaucratic burden), the JD-R framework opens up two paths for intervention. It invites decision-makers to reduce hindering demands that are not relevant to fulfil the teaching duty and to support the complexities of core teaching tasks by providing adequate resources. Job resources refer to the 'physical, psychological, social or organizational aspects of the job that have motivating potential' (Demerouti et al., 2001, p. 501). These encompass elements such as pay, autonomy, social support, constructive feedback, and opportunities for growth. The model also recognizes the role of personal resources, such as self-efficacy, optimism, and professional knowledge, that help individuals navigate workplace demands (Bakker et al., 2023).

The JD-R model explains how these two forces operate in parallel: High demands can lead to burnout and strain, while sufficient resources can protect against this deterioration and actively fuel commitment and satisfaction. When applied to the educational context, this model provides a clear rationale for how teacher well-being is the outcome of how well systems are designed to balance these opposing forces (Fig. 3). What makes the JD-R model especially valuable for policymaking is its ability to trace outcomes back to upstream decisions. Many of the job demands teachers face – for example, teaching hours, workload, and class sizes – are direct consequences of policy decisions. Likewise, many of the resources that could mitigate these

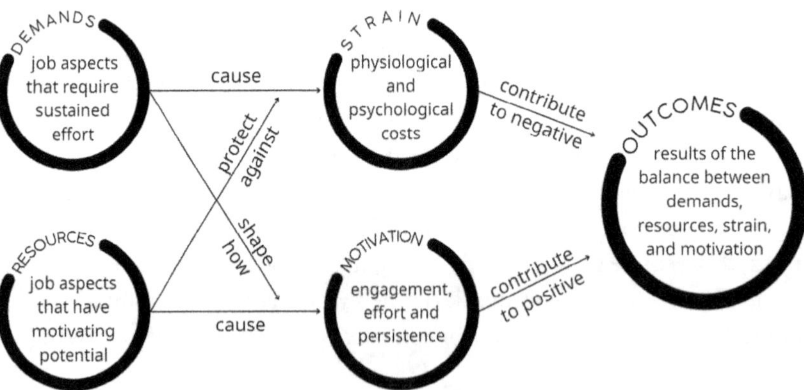

Fig. 3. Job Demands–Resources Model by Demerouti et al. (2001). Figure Created by the Author.

pressures – for example, autonomy, time for collaboration, access to professional development, and stable leadership – are made possible only through thoughtful structural planning. In this way, the model offers a conceptual bridge between policy levers and lived experiences.

Furthermore, the JD-R framework is not only diagnostic but also action-oriented. It enables a shift from reactive responses, such as burnout interventions or isolated wellness programmes, to proactive strategies that address root causes. It makes visible the mechanics of how resources become most effective precisely when demands are high, suggesting that investment in support mechanisms should be aligned with the intensity of job requirements. It also reinforces the importance of coherence across levels; a policy promoting autonomy, for instance, will only be successful if it is echoed in school leadership practices and trusted by teams (Bakker et al., 2023). In this light, the JD-R model aids policymakers in identifying where breakdowns in teacher well-being originate, how those problems manifest across different levels of the system, and where leverage exists to create meaningful change.

The following subsections gather evidence about what policies can change or prioritize with respect to teacher well-being. By means of the JD-R model, these are divided into measures to reduce hindering demands and measures to increase resources for tackling the inherent demands of teaching. The following suggestions are grounded in JD-R theory and current research findings. If certain aspects appear to be missing, it may be due to a lack of empirical investigation or inconclusive evidence regarding their effectiveness.

3.1. REDUCE HINDERING DEMANDS

3.1.1. Class Size

Smaller class sizes have been associated with improvements in teacher well-being across various studies. Indicators such as job satisfaction, professional morale, and perceived workload appear positively influenced when teachers are responsible for fewer students. Evidence suggests that teaching in classrooms with fewer than 20 students is linked to lower stress levels, particularly in relation to addressing individual student needs and managing classroom dynamics. In contrast, larger classes are often perceived as more stressful and demanding, with adverse implications for mental health and instructional quality.

Research indicates that smaller classes reduce the intensity and breadth of the workload, enabling teachers to allocate their time more effectively, engage in higher quality instruction, and experience a stronger sense of professional efficacy. These conditions contribute to greater job satisfaction and overall well-being. Additionally, reduced class sizes are frequently associated with improved classroom management and the ability to provide more individualized attention, which in turn enhances the teaching experience.

> Literature reviewed: N. French, 1993; Hojo, 2021; Karjalainen et al., 2020; W. Price & Terry, 2008; M. L. Smith & Glass, 1980; Undie & Nike, 2016.

3.1.1.1. Measure

Implement sensible, context-sensitive class size limits.

3.1.1.1.1. 3 Key Components

- **Set evidence-based maximum class size thresholds**

  Establish class size limits grounded in empirical research on student learning and teacher workload. These thresholds should reflect the developmental stages of students and the pedagogical demands of different subjects.

- **Link limits to staffing and infrastructure planning**

  Ensure that class size policies are supported by adequate teacher recruitment, classroom space, and learning resources. This includes forward-looking infrastructure planning to prevent unintended overcrowding in other classes.

- **Prioritize implementation in high-need contexts**

  Apply class size limits first in schools experiencing high workload stress, persistent teacher shortages, or low student achievement. Special attention should be given to disadvantaged communities to ensure equitable access to supportive learning environments.

For Measure Dashboard, see Table 1.

3.1.1.2. Good-Practice Examples[1]

3.1.1.2.1. Japan: Primary School Class Size Limited to 35 Students. In 2021, the Japanese Government (Ministry of Education, Culture, Sports, Science and Technology, MEXT) formally lowered the maximum class size in primary

1 Please note: Most good-practice examples in this book reflect progress within a specific context, not universally impressive solutions. What seems modest in one setting may be a significant achievement elsewhere, depending on local challenges and constraints.

Table 1. Measure Dashboard for Class Size.

Dimension	Rating	Description
Impact	●●● **High**	Strong potential to transform teacher well-being. Addresses key drivers and has broad, lasting impact
Quality of Evidence	●●○ **Moderate**	Some research support, possibly from case studies or correlational data. Promising but not conclusive
Context Dependency	●●○ **Moderate**	Requires some adaptation but can function in several settings; effectiveness depends on moderately specific conditions (e.g. type of school)
Sustainability	●●○ **High**	Embedded in institutional routines or culture; self-sustaining with minimal additional support
Teacher Voice	●●○ **Low**	Teachers have little or no input; top-down implementation
Implementation Feasibility	●●○ **Low**	Difficult to implement; requires substantial time, resources, training, or systemic change. Often needs external support or policy alignment

schools from 40 to 35 students (Hojo, 2021). This change, as part of Japan's Basic Plan for Education Promotion, was explicitly aimed at easing teachers' excessive workloads and stress (Japan has some of the longest teacher working hours in OECD data). A recent analysis of Japanese Teaching and Learning International Survey (TALIS) data found that high student–teacher ratios were significantly associated with longer teacher working hours and increased stress, and that reducing a class by five students cut weekly teacher work by approximately 2.8 hours. The author concluded that the 2021 class size reduction policy 'could reduce teacher stress and long work hours' (p. 2). The implementation required hiring additional teachers to fill the smaller classes.

3.1.1.2.2. Estonia: City Enacts Class Size Limit of 24 Students. In 2023 to 2025, the city of Tallinn moved to enforce the national class size cap of 24 students by limiting first-grade intake. The Tallinn City Council drafted regulations (approved February 2025) to cap new Grade 1 classes at 24 students each (Tallinn City Government, 2025). Tallinn's mayor explained that the goal is twofold: 'children can learn in smaller classes' and 'teachers can work with a manageable workload' (para. 2). Tallinn had over 700 existing classes with more than 24 students (2,000+ students), which 'places additional strain on teachers' (para. 5). By creating new school places and enforcing the 24-student limit (starting with Grade 1 in September 2025), the policy aims to relieve overcrowding and reduce teacher overload over time. This city-level case is notable because the rationale explicitly addresses teacher workload and well-being; it is currently being rolled out and will be evaluated in the coming years.

3.1.2. Workload and Time Pressure

Teacher workload, spanning instructional responsibilities, administrative tasks, and extracurricular obligations, has been consistently associated with diminished well-being outcomes across diverse educational settings. High workloads are linked to increased stress, emotional exhaustion, burnout, anxiety, and depression, as well as lower levels of job satisfaction and professional engagement.

Multiple studies across different countries report that teachers frequently cite workload as a primary contributor to psychological strain. Among the various components of workload, administrative duties are often viewed as particularly burdensome, as they tend to reduce perceived professional autonomy and add layers of complexity that detract from core teaching activities.

Evidence suggests that noninstructional tasks such as reporting, data entry, and compliance procedures may be more predictive of burnout than classroom-related duties. While teaching itself is demanding, many educators perceive direct instruction and student engagement as meaningful and intrinsically rewarding. In contrast, administrative demands are typically experienced as misaligned with the core purpose of teaching, leading to frustration and fatigue.

Several moderating variables influence the relationship between workload and well-being. Organizational factors, such as leadership support, collegial relationships, and school climate, can buffer the negative effects of high demands. Individual-level characteristics, including emotion regulation capacity, perceived self-efficacy, and preparedness through training, also appear to play a protective role. Importantly, early-career teachers and those experiencing disproportionate administrative responsibilities are identified as particularly vulnerable to the adverse effects of excessive workload.

These findings underscore that the quantity and type of workload are not merely logistical challenges but are closely linked to teachers' physical and psychological health. The nature of these tasks and the degree to which they align with teachers' professional identity and values play a significant role in determining their impact. Accordingly, interventions targeting teacher well-being must address structural factors such as workload distribution, task relevance, and autonomy in task execution. Systemic change, rather than individual coping alone, is necessary to mitigate workload-related stress and to support teacher retention and thriving in the profession.

Literature reviewed: Carroll et al., 2022; Jellis et al., 2021; Kidger et al., 2016; Lawrence et al., 2018; Naghieh et al., 2015; Ortan et al., 2021; Pan et al., 2023; Skinner et al., 2019; Timms et al., 2007.

3.1.2.1. Measure

Implement comprehensive workload regulations that reduce administrative burden, protect instructional time, and align teachers' responsibilities with their core professional roles.

3.1.2.1.1. 3 Key Components

- **Establish clear guidelines to limit noninstructional duties**

  Develop national or regional regulations that restrict excessive administrative requirements, such as data reporting, compliance paperwork, and bureaucratic documentation. These guidelines should ensure that teachers' time is prioritized for teaching and student support.

- **Strengthen administrative support structures in schools**

  Allocate funding to hire and train school-based administrative staff who can assume routine nonteaching responsibilities. This investment allows teachers to focus on instruction while ensuring necessary administrative tasks are handled efficiently.

- **Protect planning time and support vulnerable groups**

  Mandate dedicated hours within the school schedule for lesson preparation, professional reflection, and peer collaboration. Early-career teachers and those with disproportionate administrative responsibilities should receive additional protections to mitigate their vulnerability to excessive workload pressures.

For Measure Dashboard, see Table 2.

3.1.2.2. Good-Practice Examples

3.1.2.2.1. Philippines: National Policy on Teacher Workload Allocation. In 2024, the Philippine Department of Education issued DepEd Order No. 5, s. 2024, a nationwide policy designed to structure and limit teachers' workload by clearly distinguishing between instructional and ancillary duties. Under this order, public school teachers are allocated 6 hours of daily teaching

Table 2. Measure Dashboard for Workload.

Dimension	Rating	Description
Impact	●●● **High**	Strong potential to transform teacher well-being. Addresses key drivers and has broad, lasting impact
Quality of Evidence	●●● **High**	Strong, consistent evidence from rigorous research (e.g. meta-analyses, randomized controlled trials, longitudinal studies). Widely accepted in the field
Context Dependency	●○○ **Low**	Works effectively across most educational settings with minimal or no adaptation; broadly transferable
Sustainability	●●● **High**	Embedded in institutional routines or culture; self-sustaining with minimal additional support
Teacher Voice	●○○ **Low**	Teachers have little or no input; top-down implementation
Implementation Feasibility	●○○ **Low**	Difficult to implement; requires substantial time, resources, training, or systemic change. Often needs external support or policy alignment

and 2 hours for essential nonteaching tasks, such as lesson planning, grading, and student support.

The policy addresses longstanding concerns about teacher overload by

- prioritizing core teaching responsibilities,
- regulating overtime: allowing extra hours only in cases of teacher shortages and requiring either compensation or service credits, and
- promoting transparency and accountability through required documentation, monitoring, and reporting mechanisms.

This structured approach helps ensure that teacher time is managed fairly and realistically, which is crucial in a system where administrative overload has been a major contributor to stress and burnout. A study by Zerna (2025) gathered teacher feedback on the policy's early implementation. While most teachers welcomed the initiative as well-intentioned, they emphasized that its success depends heavily on consistent enforcement, adequate staffing, and supportive school leadership. When these conditions are met, the policy holds significant promise for improving teacher well-being and retention.

3.1.2.2.2. United States: 4-Day Teacher Week to Improve Workload Balance. In Jefferson County, Colorado, education leaders responded to rising concerns about teacher burnout, workload, and retention by introducing a district-wide 4-day school week (Y.-J. Yu, 2023). Under the new policy, students attend from Tuesday to Friday, while Mondays are reserved for teacher use. The policy was designed with two objectives: to improve teacher work–life balance and to strengthen recruitment and retention. A veteran teacher described the immediate impact: 'When I start on Tuesday, I really feel far more prepared than I ever did on the five-day week' (para. 3). Crucially, the district ensured that Mondays were not lost instructional time but were strategically used for professional development. As the superintendent explained, 'We have our teachers come in ... one Monday a month, a half day in the mornings and do all their professional development. This approach balanced flexibility with system-wide consistency' (para. 12).

The results illustrate how workload-focused policy shifts can pay dividends. Teacher morale improved, and the reform directly addressed chronic staffing challenges. Applications for open positions increased to '10 to 12 candidates' (para. 16) per role – compared to only a handful before the change. Administrators reported being 'fully staffed' for the first time in years, highlighting the effectiveness of the reform in strengthening the teacher pipeline.

3.2. INCREASE RESOURCES

3.2.1. Quality Teacher Education

Research suggests that a strong grounding in content knowledge and pedagogical expertise is the bedrock of effective teaching and plays a critical role in teacher well-being. Teachers who feel confident in what they teach and how they teach it experience greater self-efficacy, job satisfaction, and a stronger professional identity. They are more likely to see their work as meaningful, which buffers against burnout and emotional exhaustion. When teachers possess solid instructional competencies, they are not constantly operating in survival mode, Instead, they are able to focus on deeper engagement with students and the curriculum, reinforcing their sense of purpose and professional fulfilment.

Among the core professional skills, effective classroom management stands out as one of the most influential contributors to teacher well-being. Teachers who lack the tools to manage behaviour constructively often report high levels of stress, emotional exhaustion, and even feelings of professional failure. In contrast, proactive and structured classroom management strategies are strongly associated with lower stress levels, improved student behaviour, and enhanced teacher morale. Importantly, these strategies empower teachers to feel in control of their classrooms, contributing to a sense of agency and reducing psychological strain. Closely connected to management abilities is the teacher's social and emotional competence. Teaching is an emotionally demanding profession, and those with strong emotional regulation, relational skills, and self-awareness are better equipped to maintain supportive relationships, de-escalate conflict, and foster emotionally safe classroom environments.

However, long-term teacher well-being depends not only on what is taught in teacher education but also on how teacher education is structured. Evidence suggests that systematic, practice-oriented preparation is essential to prevent the so-called Praxisschock – the disillusionment and stress that arise when new teachers first confront the unpredictable, emotionally taxing realities of the classroom. Well-designed teacher education programmes gradually increase in complexity and integrate extensive, supervised practicum experiences. These provide authentic exposure to real classroom challenges while allowing time for reflection, guided feedback, and peer support. Such scaffolding prepares candidates for the emotional and logistical demands of teaching and helps them build confidence before entering the profession. Structured mentoring and coaching during the early years of teaching are critical buffers against stress and burnout. These relationships provide emotional reassurance, practical advice, and a sense of belonging, all of which are central to sustaining motivation and preventing early attrition.

In addition to these more general aspects, there is a growing case for including dedicated courses on teacher well-being. These courses legitimize the emotional dimensions of the profession, helping future teachers understand that stress and vulnerability are normal, not signs of weakness. They also equip teachers with concrete tools for emotional self-regulation, such as cognitive–behavioural techniques, mindfulness strategies, and reflective practices that can be applied throughout their careers. Perhaps most importantly, such courses foster a proactive mindset, encouraging teachers to recognize early warning signs of psychological strain in themselves and others and to seek or offer support. This contributes to a more sustainable, compassionate professional culture.

Literature reviewed: Clunies-Ross et al., 2008; Eloff & Dittrich, 2021; Jennings & Greenberg, 2009; Kennedy et al., 2021; Korthagen et al., 2001; Lauth-Lebens & Lauth, 2016; Leckey et al., 2016; Marlow et al., 2015; Nazari & Karimpour, 2024; Wu et al., 2022; Zee & Koomen, 2016.

3.2.1.1. Measure

Ensure the quality of teacher education and a focus on teacher well-being.

3.2.1.1.1. 3 Key Components

- **Mandate the integration of core professional competencies**

  Strengthen the inclusion of comprehensive training in content knowledge, pedagogical skill, classroom management, and social–emotional competence.

- **Advance the design of practice-based learning**

  Ensure that teacher education curricula include practicum phases that include meaningful, supervised teaching experiences. These should be supported by structured mentoring systems that provide emotional support, feedback, and guidance during both initial training and early-career stages.

- **Promote the inclusion of dedicated courses on teacher well-being**

  Introduce dedicated courses that address teacher well-being explicitly. Courses must be research backed and tailored to the teaching profession.

For Measure Dashboard, see Table 3.

Table 3. Measure Dashboard for Quality Teacher Education.

Dimension	Rating	Description
Impact	●●● **High**	Strong potential to transform teacher well-being. Addresses key drivers and has a broad, lasting impact
Quality of Evidence	●●● **High**	Strong, consistent evidence from rigorous research (e.g. meta-analyses, randomized controlled trials, longitudinal studies). Widely accepted in the field
Context Dependency	●●○ **Moderate**	Requires some adaptation but can function in several settings; effectiveness depends on moderately specific conditions (e.g. type of school).
Sustainability	●●● **High**	Embedded in institutional routines or culture; self-sustaining with minimal additional support
Teacher Voice	●●○ **Moderate**	Some consultation with teachers, but limited decision-making power
Implementation Feasibility	●●○ **Moderate**	Requires some planning, adjustment, or collaboration. Feasible with committed leadership and moderate resource input

3.2.1.2. Good-Practice Examples

3.2.1.2.1. England: National Framework Embedding Well-Being in Teacher Training. The UK government introduced a new Initial Teacher Training (ITT) Core Content Framework (alongside the Early Career Framework) that explicitly requires teacher educators to train future teachers in managing workload and self-care. This includes that 'trainees should be supported to manage their own workload and well-being whilst they train and as they embark on their career in school' (Department for Education, 2024, p. 7). For example, teacher candidates are expected to 'learn how to manage workload and wellbeing' by:

- observing how experienced colleagues apply and adapt systems and routines for effective time and task management and critically reflecting on these practices;
- engaging in professional dialogue with expert colleagues to analyze the importance of accessing appropriate support – such as when addressing student misbehaviour;
- recognizing the value of protecting time for rest and recovery, and developing awareness of available resources that promote and sustain good mental health. (pp. 30–31)

3.2.1.2.2. Scotland: Nationwide Resilience and Well-Being Programme in Teacher Development. Education Scotland launched the nationwide Resilience and Well-being Series for Educators, a professional development programme for teachers. This 8- to 12-hr webinar series trains teachers in psychological resilience. Participants learn how their minds handle stress and acquire tools to manage anxiety, work–life balance, and workload. Its stated aim is to help educators 'uncover their own inbuilt capacity for mental health and wellbeing thus enhancing their capacity and potential to deal more effectively with personal and professional challenges and be more impactful in their role' (Education Scotland, 2025, para. 1).

3.2.2. Pay

Pay is a considerable factor in teacher well-being. When teachers are underpaid or face financial insecurity, their well-being suffers, their stress levels rise, and their desire to leave the profession intensifies. This link is especially pronounced in low-income or crisis-affected contexts, where pay is not just a matter of satisfaction. In these settings, competitive and timely compensation can be the difference between retention and attrition, with effects primarily operating through teacher well-being.

Yet, the evidence also tells a more layered story. In contexts where basic financial needs are met, psychological and organizational factors, such as autonomy, professional growth, and school climate, take centre stage. What matters most, then, is context. In environments marked by financial hardship, salary becomes a frontline issue. In more stable settings, the broader ecology of support plays a defining role. However, perceived fairness (e.g. with comparable jobs or between different school types) in pay remains an important issue.

Literature reviewed: Assaf & Antoun, 2024; Bullough et al., 2012; Kingdon, 2010; J. Liu, 2020; McQuade, 2024; Naghieh et al., 2015; Song et al., 2020; Tang et al., 2018; Yuan et al., 2013.

3.2.2.1. Measure

Guarantee competitive, fair, reliable, and context-appropriate teacher pay, particularly in low-income or crisis-affected settings.

3.2.2.1.1. 3 Key Components

- **Regularly benchmark teacher salaries**

  Align teacher pay with the local cost of living, inflation, and salaries in comparable professions to maintain financial stability and professional recognition.

- **Introduce targeted financial incentives in high-need contexts**

  Provide pay premiums or hardship allowances in disadvantaged or fragile areas where financial stress most strongly affects teacher well-being and retention.

- **Establish transparent monitoring systems**

  Develop mechanisms to track the impact of pay structures on teacher satisfaction, well-being, and attrition. Data should be disaggregated by region, gender, and school type to support equitable outcomes and policy refinement.

For Measure Dashboard, see Table 4.

Table 4. Measure Dashboard 04 for Pay.

Dimension	Rating	Description
Impact	●●○ **Moderate**	Has a noticeable effect for some contexts or groups. Contributes meaningfully but not comprehensively
Quality of Evidence	●●● **High**	Strong, consistent evidence from rigorous research (e.g. meta-analyses, randomized controlled trials, longitudinal studies). Widely accepted in the field
Context Dependency	●●● **High**	Highly dependent on specific cultural, institutional, or socioeconomic contexts; effectiveness is limited outside of these
Sustainability	●●○ **Moderate**	Some integration into structures or culture but still somewhat dependent on leadership or budget
Teacher Voice	●○○ **Low**	Teachers have little or no input; top-down implementation
Implementation Feasibility	●○○ **Low**	Difficult to implement; requires substantial time, resources, training, or systemic change. Often needs external support or policy alignment

3.2.2.2. Good-Practice Examples

3.2.2.2.1. Afghanistan: Introduction of Mobile Salary Payments. From 2017 to 2020, the Afghan government (with World Bank support) rolled out a Mobile Salary Payment (MSP) reform. All Ministry of Education staff (teachers and principals) were biometrically registered and paid via mobile money accounts instead of cash. This aimed to eliminate 'ghost' teachers and reduce chronic delays and leakages in pay. An evaluation found that transitioning teachers to a biometric registration and mobile money system significantly improved their overall satisfaction, particularly by reducing longstanding issues with salary delays (Blumenstock et al., 2023). While the reform did not fully eliminate ghost workers or drastically reduce payment leakage, it led to substantial improvements in the payment experience. Delays dropped from affecting over half of teachers to just 30%, with the most notable improvements in urban areas. In addition to increasing financial inclusion, the reform also correlated with improved student learning outcomes in cities, suggesting that better and more timely compensation may have boosted teacher morale and effectiveness.

3.2.2.2.2. Hungary: National Teacher Pay Increase and Performance-Based Raises. The Hungarian government implemented a 32% average salary increase in 2024, with an additional 20% to 21% raise planned for 2025, aiming to bring average teacher salaries to roughly 80% of graduate-level earnings. Disadvantaged areas receive a further 20% premium, and shortage-posted teachers receive an extra 7% allowance. Performance evaluation now factors into future raises, shifting away from purely seniority-based increases (MTI-Hungary Today, 2023).

3.2.3. School Autonomy

School autonomy is associated with enhanced well-being among both teachers and students, though the strength and nature of these effects vary according to contextual and measurement factors. Teachers who report greater instructional autonomy or involvement in decision-making processes tend to experience higher job satisfaction, greater engagement, and reduced levels of stress and emotional exhaustion. For students, perceptions of teacher autonomy support are linked with increased school satisfaction, enjoyment, and self-rated health, although associations with social integration appear more variable.

Cross-national evidence suggests that autonomy tends to yield more positive outcomes in education systems with strong institutional support and regulatory capacity. In contrast, the benefits of autonomy may be weaker or less consistent in underresourced or structurally unstable contexts. Moderating and mediating variables, such as school size, teacher self-efficacy, intrinsic motivation, and workload significantly shape how autonomy translates into well-being outcomes.

Overall, findings indicate that autonomy is not inherently beneficial or harmful, but its impact is contingent upon the broader organizational and cultural conditions in which it is implemented. When embedded within supportive and well-functioning environments, autonomy can serve as a powerful lever for improving both teacher and student well-being.

Literature reviewed: Hanushek et al., 2012; Kleinkorres et al., 2023; Lima et al., 2024; Nie et al., 2014; Paletta, 2014; Pan et al., 2023; Skaalvik & Skaalvik, 2014; Wößmann, 2007.

3.2.3.1. Measure

Ensure meaningful, context-sensitive school autonomy, particularly in instructional decision-making and participatory governance.

3.2.3.1.1. 3 Key Components

- **Establish inclusive school-level decision-making bodies**

  Mandate councils or committees that include teachers and other staff to participate in curriculum planning, resource allocation, and professional development priorities.

- **Provide flexibility in instructional approaches**

  Provide schools and teachers with adequate flexibility in selecting instructional methods and classroom strategies, tailored to student needs, while maintaining clear outcome-based accountability (e.g. via student learning benchmarks rather than prescriptive methods).

- **Implement differentiated autonomy policies**

  Develop differentiated autonomy policies based on local conditions. For instance, schools in high-need or underresourced areas receive additional leadership training, mentorship structures, and reduced administrative burden to ensure autonomy does not translate into unmanaged responsibility or inequity.

For Measure Dashboard, see Table 5.

Table 5. Measure Dashboard for School Autonomy.

Dimension	Rating	Description
Impact	●●○ **Moderate**	Has a noticeable effect for some contexts or groups. Contributes meaningfully but not comprehensively
Quality of Evidence	●●○ **Moderate**	Some research support possibly from case studies or correlational data. Promising but not conclusive
Context Dependency	●●○ **Moderate**	Requires some adaptation but can function in several settings; effectiveness depends on moderately specific conditions (e.g. type of school).
Sustainability	●●○ **Moderate**	Some integration into structures or culture, but still somewhat dependent on leadership or budget
Teacher Voice	●○○ **Low**	Teachers have little or no input; top-down implementation
Implementation Feasibility	●●○ **Moderate**	Requires some planning, adjustment, or collaboration. Feasible with committed leadership and moderate resource input

3.2.3.2. Good-Practice Examples

3.2.3.2.1. England: National Extension of Flexible Working Ambassadors Programme. In May 2025, the UK Department for Education announced a national extension of its Flexible Working Ambassadors Programme, resulting in 46% of state school teachers now enjoying formal flexible working arrangements, a six percentage point rise since 2022 (Department for Education, 2025). The initiative enables teachers to undertake tasks such as lesson planning, marking, and job-sharing outside classroom hours, with the aim of reducing workload stress and improving retention. Government data show that 47% of teachers considering leaving cited insufficient flexibility as a key issue, while 82% of school leaders offering flexible arrangements agreed it helped retain staff. The policy is positioned within a broader strategy to recruit 6,500 expert teachers and strengthen workforce stability.

3.2.3.2.2. Wales: National Curriculum Update. Starting in 2022, Wales implemented a new statutory national curriculum defined by the Curriculum and Assessment (Wales) Act 2021. This reform empowers schools to develop their own curricula within a framework of six Areas of Learning and Experience. Rather than prescribing specific content or timelines, schools determine what and how they teach, promoting flexibility in pedagogy and integration across subjects (e.g. digital competence, health, and well-being). Initial surveys report broad teacher support for increased professional responsibility and relevance of content, although some express challenges around clarity and resource alignment (Wightwick 2022).

3.2.3.2.3. Portugal: Autonomy and Curricular Flexibility Project. Under Decree-Laws 54/2018 and 55/2018, Portugal granted participating schools the autonomy to manage up to 25% of curriculum time, enabling them to tailor content to local needs and adopt inclusive or innovative teaching approaches. This formal policy followed pilot initiatives from 2016 to 2018 that were designed to promote inclusion and pedagogical innovation. The rationale was to reduce school failure, boost teaching quality, and give schools the power to adjust programmes contextually without altering national standards. Evaluations indicate that many educators welcomed the increased pedagogical freedom, which allowed them to better adapt their teaching to diverse student needs and foster a stronger sense of professional purpose aligned with inclusive education values (OECD, 2022).

In supportive school environments, this autonomy also enhanced collaboration and innovation among staff. However, the OECD also found that these benefits were unevenly experienced. Many teachers felt underprepared for the demands of inclusive teaching, citing limited practical training, unclear roles, and burdensome professional development obligations. Additionally, systemic constraints, such as centralized hiring, unstable contracts, and a lack of time and resources, often undermined the well-being gains that greater autonomy was meant to deliver.

3.2.4. Systemic Appreciation

Emerging research suggests that appreciation – that is, being seen, recognized, and acknowledged for one's efforts – is a powerful contributor to teacher well-being. Conversely, the absence of appreciation, especially in environments marked by increasing demands and public scrutiny, can erode morale and deepen stress.

Interviews with teachers during the COVID-19 pandemic illustrate this vividly. At first, as families experienced the challenges of homeschooling, appreciation for teachers surged. Parents expressed gratitude for the work teachers were doing under extraordinary circumstances. But over time, that sentiment faded. As expectations increased and understanding waned, teachers began to feel invisible again, reporting not only a loss of public recognition but also a deepened sense of emotional strain.

Large-scale studies show that teachers who feel genuinely appreciated – especially by students, colleagues, and school leaders – report higher job satisfaction, lower emotional exhaustion, and a reduced likelihood of leaving the profession. Consistent, everyday recognition within their immediate work environment has the strongest impact. Appreciation from society and policymakers also contributes, though more indirectly: Positive public discourse reinforces professional pride and legitimacy, while negative or absent recognition can erode collective morale and exacerbate burnout, particularly under high workload conditions.

Literature reviewed: Allen et al., 2024; Ashiedu & Scott-Ladd, 2012; Carlo et al., 2013; Dreer-Goethe, 2025b; L. E. Kim et al., 2024; Pfister, 2019; Pfister et al., 2020; Spruyt et al., 2021; Stocker et al., 2014.

3.2.4.1. Measure

Integrate consistent and meaningful appreciation into education policy, emphasizing recognition from students, parents, and school communities.

3.2.4.1.1. 3 Key Components

- **Implement recurring appreciation campaigns**

  Develop national or regional campaigns co-created with educators to ensure recognition is authentic, meaningful, and avoids tokenism.

- **Embed teacher recognition in official communications**

  Incorporate acknowledgment of teacher contributions into ministry communications, public events, and formal award systems.

- **Promote public acknowledgment by education authorities**

  Encourage school and district leaders to regularly recognize teacher efforts, reinforcing professional respect and morale.

For Measure Dashboard, see Table 6.

3.2.4.2. Good-Practice Examples

3.2.4.2.1. Australia: Be That Teacher National Status-Raising Campaign. In October 2023, the federal government launched the Be That Teacher national

Table 6. Measure Dashboard for Appreciation.

Dimension	Rating	Description
Impact	●●○ **Moderate**	Has a noticeable effect for some contexts or groups. Contributes meaningfully but not comprehensively
Quality of Evidence	●●○ **Moderate**	Some research support, possibly from case studies or correlational data. Promising but not conclusive
Context Dependency	●●○ **Moderate**	Requires some adaptation but can function in several settings; effectiveness depends on moderately specific conditions (e.g. type of school)
Sustainability	●●○ **Moderate**	Some integration into structures or culture, but still somewhat dependent on leadership or budget
Teacher Voice	●○○ **Low**	Teachers have little or no input; top-down implementation
Implementation Feasibility	●●● **High**	Easy to implement; minimal resources or barriers. Can be adopted with little disruption to daily practice

media campaign (Department for Education, 2023). This symbolic initiative features real teacher stories on TV, billboards, and social media to raise the status of the teaching profession and encourage more people to consider teaching. Its goal is to improve public respect for teachers and to help recruit more high-calibre candidates.

3.2.4.2.2. Bangladesh: National Teacher Celebration and Welfare Trust Programme. The Bangladeshi government institutionalized World Teachers' Day (5 October) as a national event in 2023 (following its first celebration in 2022). High-profile ceremonies now celebrate teachers' contributions and confer awards. Officials emphasize showing 'respect and gratitude to the honourable teachers' as a way to 'attract younger generations to join the teaching profession' and 'elevating the status of teachers' (UNESCO, 2023, para. 7).

3.2.4.2.3. Indonesia: Government-Supported Teacher Housing Scheme. In early 2025, the Ministry of Primary and Secondary Education and the Ministry of Housing and Residential Areas began handing over subsidized homes to teachers. The pilot transfer of keys (250 units, with ~20,000 planned) targets low-income public teachers. The policy aims to improve teacher well-being and ensure teachers live near their schools, so they can 'focus more on supporting students' learning' (Kenzu, 2025, para. 5). Officials call teachers 'heroes of national education' whose welfare should be improved (Kenzu, 2025, para. 9).

3.2.5. Supportive Leadership

Research consistently demonstrates that supportive leadership plays a crucial role in enhancing teacher well-being and overall school effectiveness. Transformational and positive leadership styles are particularly effective in fostering teacher well-being. School leaders can improve teacher well-being by creating a positive school culture, providing meaningful professional development and involving teachers in decision-making processes. Supportive leadership is associated with higher levels of teacher well-being, job satisfaction, and willingness to promote their schools. During crises like the COVID-19 pandemic, distributed and compassionate leadership styles are particularly beneficial for supporting teacher well-being. The relationship between teacher leadership and well-being is reciprocal, with each positively influencing the other. Recent bibliometric analysis confirms the growing research interest in this field and the consistent emphasis on leadership's impact on teacher well-being.

Literature reviewed: Cann et al., 2020; Cherkowski, 2018; Ghamrawi et al., 2023; Karakus, Toprak, & Chen, 2024; Kwatubana & Molaodi, 2021; M. H. Lee & Swaner, 2023; Meidelina et al., 2023; Venema-Steen et al., 2023.

3.2.5.1. Measure

Make supportive leadership for teacher well-being a core requirement in school leadership standards and evaluation.

3.2.5.1.1. 3 Key Components

- **Mandate certified leadership training**

  Require all current and aspiring principals and school leaders to complete certified professional development in transformational, distributed, and compassionate leadership, with specific modules on supporting teacher well-being and managing staff during crises.

- **Include teacher well-being indicators in leadership performance reviews**

  Embed specific, evidence-based indicators of teacher well-being (e.g. staff retention, survey data, satisfaction rates, qualitative feedback) into school leader performance evaluations. Make sustained improvements in staff well-being a criterion for advancement or renewal.

- **Implement annual teacher well-being audits**

  Mandate an annual, anonymous teacher well-being audit in every school. Survey results must be reviewed by leadership teams and school boards and used to create targeted improvement actions tied to school planning and leadership evaluations.

For Measure Dashboard, see Table 7.

3.2.5.2. Good-Practice Example

3.2.5.2.1. Australia and Aotearoa New Zealand: National Leadership Standards and Well-Being Focus. In Australia and Aotearoa New Zealand, government-backed leadership frameworks emphasize a positive school culture and teacher support. Australia's national Professional Standard for Principals (Australian Institute for Teaching and School Leadership [AITSL]) requires school leaders to 'create a positive culture of challenge and support' (AITSL,

Table 7. Measure Dashboard for Supportive Leadership.

Dimension	Rating	Description
Impact	●●● **High**	Strong potential to transform teacher well-being. Addresses key drivers and has a broad, lasting impact
Quality of Evidence	●●● **High**	Strong, consistent evidence from rigorous research (e.g. meta-analyses, randomized controlled trials, longitudinal studies). Widely accepted in the field
Context Dependency	●○○ **Low**	Works effectively across most educational settings with minimal or no adaptation; broadly transferable
Sustainability	●●○ **Moderate**	Some integration into structures or culture, but still somewhat dependent on leadership or budget
Teacher Voice	●●● **High**	Teachers co-design, adapt, and lead the initiative; their professional knowledge is central
Implementation Feasibility	●●○ **Moderate**	Requires some planning, adjustment, or collaboration. Feasible with committed leadership and moderate resource input

2014, p. 12) for effective teaching. The standard also calls for building trust, collaboration, and mentoring cultures within schools. Teacher–leader professional learning is high priority: The Australian Government has funded principal development programmes that include modules on staff well-being and engagement, recognizing that leader behaviour is critical for a healthy work environment. Outcomes are evaluated via principal surveys (AITSL), showing supportive leadership practices are linked to teacher retention.

In Aotearoa New Zealand, the Education Council's Educational Leadership Capability Framework and Leadership Strategy for the Teaching Profession emphasize principals' well-being and their role in supporting staff well-being (New Zealand Council for Educational Research, 2018). For example, one core competency is 'attending to their own learning as leaders and their own wellbeing' (p. 6), promoting self-care. The framework also highlights leaders' responsibility to 'contribute to the development and wellbeing of education' beyond their own school (p. 7). While not mandatory, the Teaching Council provides toolkits and case studies to help principals support teacher well-being.

3.2.6. Well-Being Programmes

Research indicates that teacher supervision, mentoring, coaching, and intervention programmes can significantly improve teacher well-being. For example, mindfulness training has been shown to reduce stress, anxiety, depression, and burnout while increasing mindfulness, self-compassion, and overall well-being in teachers. These benefits can be sustained long term, with continued improvements in mindfulness and self-compassion observed months after programme completion. Mindfulness practices also enhance teachers' emotion regulation, focused attention, and working memory capacity. Additionally, coaching mindset development has been found to positively impact educators' professional and personal well-being by improving relationships and increasing hope and efficacy. Implementing mindfulness and coaching programmes in teacher education and professional development may help promote well-being, prevent burnout, and improve teaching quality in schools.

Literature reviewed: Beames et al., 2022; Dave et al., 2020; Dreer & Gouasé, 2021; Dye et al., 2019; Hue & Lau, 2015; Jennings et al., 2019; Lowery, 2019; Roeser et al., 2013; Roeser et al., 2012; Zarate et al., 2019.

3.2.6.1. Measure

Integrate structured well-being programmes into all stages of the teaching profession.

3.2.6.1.1. 3 Key Components

- **Implement mandatory well-being modules in teacher education and induction**

  Ensure all preservice programmes and induction years provide structured training in well-being programmes that, while adaptable to local contexts, are evidence-based and proven to be effective.

- **Offer ongoing access to school-based mentoring, coaching, and supervision**

  Establish in-school systems where teachers receive regular, confidential support from trained mentors or professional coaches. These sessions should address diverse topics related to teacher well-being.

- **Implement national standards for funding interventions**

  Provide national-level funding and guidelines to implement and scale well-being programmes across schools, ensuring sustained access and continuity. Programmes must be research backed and tailored to school contexts.

For Measure Dashboard see Table 8.

Table 8. Measure Dashboard for Well-Being Programmes.

Dimension	Rating	Description
Impact	●●● **High**	Strong potential to transform teacher well-being. Addresses key drivers and has a broad, lasting impact
Quality of Evidence	●●● **High**	Strong, consistent evidence from rigorous research (e.g. meta-analyses, randomized controlled trials, longitudinal studies). Widely accepted in the field
Context Dependency	●○○ **Low**	Works effectively across most educational settings with minimal or no adaptation; broadly transferable
Sustainability	●●○ **Moderate**	Some integration into structures or culture, but still somewhat dependent on leadership or budget
Teacher Voice	●●○ **Moderate**	Some consultation with teachers, but limited decision-making power
Implementation Feasibility	●●○ **Moderate**	Requires some planning, adjustment, or collaboration. Feasible with committed leadership and moderate resource input

3.2.6.2. Good-Practice Example

3.2.6.2.1. Singapore: Comprehensive Leadership Support and Well-Being Programmes. In 2022, Singapore's Ministry of Education (MOE) issued directives and funded programmes to support teachers' mental health. For example, the MOE introduced a 'wellness ambassador' in every school, and trained staff officers serve as peer supporters ('listening ears'; Ministry of Education Singapore, 2022). Singapore also encourages schools to form staff well-being committees with a mental health focus and provides toolkits, workshops, and counselling hotlines. Crucially, MOE leadership instructs that schools may flexibly defer or pace new initiatives to manage teachers' workload and stress. In practice, the MOE gives schools leeway in scheduling reforms (e.g. phasing in curriculum changes) so that principals can protect staff time. This multi-pronged policy is considered effective because it embeds teacher well-being in both policy and practice, rather than leaving it to ad-hoc solutions.

3.2.7. Teaching Materials and Infrastructure

Access to adequate teaching materials and functional infrastructure is a relevant contributor to teacher well-being. When schools lack essential resources, such as clean and safe environments, reliable classroom supplies, and up-to-date technology, teachers are forced to navigate daily challenges that sap their energy, reduce motivation, and hinder professional satisfaction. In these situations, inadequate physical conditions and the absence of instructional tools do more than complicate teaching; they become persistent stressors that can severely undermine teacher morale and effectiveness. This dynamic has been clearly documented in contexts such as Indonesia, where teachers have identified poor infrastructure as a primary barrier to well-being. Similar findings in Kenya and Belgium further demonstrate that sufficient materials and facilities are closely tied to teacher commitment and student learning outcomes.

The quality of the physical work environment extends beyond visible infrastructure and includes sensory conditions, especially acoustics. Poor classroom acoustics and elevated noise levels have been shown to negatively affect teachers' health and well-being. Studies link high reverberation times and constant noise exposure to increased fatigue, diminished job satisfaction, and voice strain, which are particularly common in noisy, poorly designed classrooms. Even ventilation system noise has been associated with heightened exhaustion and vocal symptoms. Consequently, acoustic treatments, noise-reduction strategies, and educational initiatives have demonstrated positive outcomes in reducing noise, improving speech intelligibility, and enhancing both teacher and student performance. These findings underscore the importance of intentionally designed classrooms in supporting teachers' physical and emotional health.

As with salary, however, the importance of material conditions must be understood in context. In underresourced or crisis-affected education systems, functional infrastructure and the availability of teaching materials are essential. In these settings, a well-equipped and safe classroom can make a critical difference between teacher retention and attrition, with far-reaching effects on student learning. In contrast, in more stable and better-resourced systems, where basic material needs are largely met, attention shifts to the organizational environment. Here, the focus is on enhancing collegial support structures, like collaborative lesson planning, shared resource development, and professional dialogue, which have become stronger predictors of both teacher well-being and instructional quality.

Yet even in high-income contexts, the perceived fairness and adequacy of available resources remain vital. Discrepancies between schools like those with modern technology and those lacking basic supplies can breed frustration and diminish morale, especially when such inequalities exist within the same district. Ultimately, what matters most is the alignment of resources with needs. In low-resource systems, ensuring basic materials and infrastructure must be the top priority. In better-resourced environments, sustaining equitable investment, maintaining physical spaces, and strengthening collaborative practices are key to supporting teachers over the long term. Across all settings, reliable access to functional tools, supportive environments, and adequate materials forms the foundation of a motivated, resilient, and professionally fulfilled teaching workforce.

Literature reviewed: Cuyvers et al., 2011; Eysel-Gosepath et al., 2013; Hasnain, 2023; Irena & Miokołaj, 2023; Karjalainen et al., 2020; Karjalainen et al., 2022; Kristiansen et al., 2011; Mealings et al., 2024; Nordgren et al., 2021; Norlander et al., 2005; Saleh et al., 2015; Shoukat, 2024; Taborda et al., 2020; Viac & Fraser, 2020.

3.2.7.1. Measure

Ensure equitable access to quality teaching materials and infrastructure.

3.2.7.1.1. 3 Key Components

- **Establish minimum standards**

  Set and monitor minimum national standards for teaching materials, classroom infrastructure, and learning environments, including acoustics, lighting, ventilation, cleanliness, and digital access.

- **Implement needs-based and transparent resource allocation**

  Develop equitable funding formulas and resource distribution frameworks that prioritize the most disadvantaged schools or regions, using data on school infrastructure, enrolment, and socioeconomic conditions.

- **Reduce inequities**

  Ensure fair distribution of teaching materials across regions and school types to prevent morale loss in underresourced schools.

For Measure Dashboard see Table 9.

3.2.7.2. Good-Practice Examples

3.2.7.2.1. Uruguay: Plan CEIBAL (One Laptop Per Child). Uruguay's Plan 'Proyecto Conectividad Educativa de Informática Básica para el Aprendizaje en Línea' (CEIBAL; *Educational Connectivity Project for Basic IT in Online*

Table 9. Measure Dashboard for Teaching Materials and Infrastructure.

Dimension	Rating	Description
Impact	●●○ **Moderate**	Has a noticeable effect for some contexts or groups. Contributes meaningfully but not comprehensively
Quality of Evidence	●●○ **Moderate**	Some research support, possibly from case studies or correlational data. Promising but not conclusive
Context Dependency	●●● **High**	Highly dependent on specific cultural, institutional, or socioeconomic contexts; effectiveness is limited outside of these
Sustainability	●●○ **Moderate**	Some integration into structures or culture, but still somewhat dependent on leadership or budget
Teacher Voice	●○○ **Low**	Teachers have little or no input; top-down implementation
Implementation Feasibility	●●○ **Moderate**	Requires some planning, adjustment, or collaboration. Feasible with committed leadership and moderate resource input

Learning) is one of the most widely cited national policies for equitable resource distribution. Starting in 2007, the government distributed free laptops to every primary student and teacher, along with no-cost internet access everywhere (World Bank Group, 2023). CEIBAL was established by presidential decree as an independent programme, ensuring continuity across governments. Teachers received training in ICT integration and technical support for maintenance. The outcomes have been striking; within a few years, the digital divide shrank dramatically. Computer access among the poorest increased from ~6% to ~92% (World Bank Group, 2023). Crucially for teachers, CEIBAL also yielded results related to well-being; surveys and studies report improved motivation among teachers. Teachers gained confidence by using tablets and interactive lessons, and professional collaboration was spurred through online communities created by the programme (Wikipedia, 2025).

3.2.7.2.2. Chile: Educarchile portal. Chile offers a model for a teacher-oriented content platform. The Educarchile portal (https://www.educarchile.cl) is 'the digital platform with the largest teachers' community in Chile and Latin America' (Fundacion Chile, 2025). Since 2001, it has provided a vast collection of curriculum-aligned materials, learning activities, lesson plans, and interactive tools for all grade levels. Educarchile integrates official syllabus requirements and encourages teachers to collaborate; educators can download resources, share their own innovations, and discuss pedagogical methods online. By 2025, more than 60,000 teachers and school managers will have registered (Fundacion Chile, 2025). Teachers credit Educarchile with simplifying lesson preparation and providing pedagogical guidance. Its success stems from strong public–private partnership; the Ministry validates content quality, while Fundación Chile ensures technological innovation and user engagement. As a result, Chilean teachers have a well-established national repository to draw on, promoting a sense of community and continuous learning that supports teacher satisfaction.

3.2.8. Teacher Voice in Policymaking

Teacher voice in policymaking can significantly contribute to teacher well-being by increasing job satisfaction and reducing negative affect. Employee voice is identified as a crucial job resource that can mitigate the detrimental effects of work-related demands. However, teachers are often marginalized in policy design processes, creating a disconnect between policy goals and implementation challenges. Engaging educators in policy design and implementation is recommended by researchers as a way to address teacher stress and improve working conditions in a meaningful manner. Teacher well-being is influenced by relationships with leaders and colleagues, emotional work, and the balance between institutional and individual well-being. Supporting teacher self-efficacy, voice, and leadership can enhance their capacity to lead educational change. Prioritizing teacher well-being in professional development and preservice programmes can empower teachers to navigate systemic constraints and flourish professionally.

> Literature reviewed: Acton & Glasgow, 2015; Bangs & Frost, 2012; Farley & Chamberlain, 2021; Good et al., 2017; Manning et al., 2020; Margolis et al., 2014; Ostermeier et al., 2023; Teacher Task Force & UNESCO, 2023; Weiland, 2021.

3.2.8.1. Measure

Strengthen teacher voice and leadership in education policy and practice.

3.2.8.1.1. 3 Key Components

- **Establish structured mechanisms for teacher participation in policymaking**

  Mandate consultation processes where teachers provide input on proposed policies affecting curriculum, workload, and well-being.

- **Hear multiple voices**

  Include teachers from various regions, education levels, and backgrounds, alongside policymakers, researchers, union representatives, and mental health experts.

- **Set well-being as a continuous topic**

  Treat well-being not as a stand-alone initiative, but as an ongoing lens for evaluating system quality, sustainability, and equity.

For Measure Dashboard, see Table 10.

3.2.8.2. Good-Practice Examples

3.2.8.2.1. Ghana: Consultative Teacher Policy Reform. Ghana's recent education reforms illustrate extensive teacher consultation. As part of a new Teacher Education Policy, the Ministry consulted 250 teachers directly to compile a report that reflected their voices and feedback, contributing to the development of a new policy framework (Teacher Task Force & UNESCO, 2024, p. 8). Teachers from across regions participated in workshops and surveys to shape the teacher policy. Although formal evaluation is pending, this has led to a teacher policy that enjoys broad buy-in and avoids polarization. Its effectiveness comes from the genuine inclusion of teacher views in drafting policy; teachers see their suggestions (on mentoring, pay, and training) reflected in the final report.

Table 10. Measure Dashboard for Teacher Voice in Policymaking.

Dimension	Rating	Description
Impact	●●● **High**	Strong potential to transform teacher well-being. Addresses key drivers and has a broad, lasting impact
Quality of Evidence	●●○ **Moderate**	Some research support, possibly from case studies or correlational data. Promising but not conclusive
Context Dependency	●●○ **Moderate**	Requires some adaptation but can function in several settings; effectiveness depends on moderately specific conditions (e.g. type of school)
Sustainability	●○○ **Low**	Requires ongoing external input or funding; unlikely to persist without constant support
Teacher Voice	●●● **High**	Teachers co-design, adapt, and lead the initiative; their professional knowledge is central
Implementation Feasibility	●●○ **Moderate**	Requires some planning, adjustment, or collaboration. Feasible with committed leadership and moderate resource input

3.2.8.2.2. Morocco: Collective Bargaining for Teacher Conditions. In 2019, the Moroccan government negotiated with major teacher unions to resolve disputes over pay and contract status. Education International reports that as a result of these talks, 'teacher working conditions and the status of contract teachers were improved' (Teacher Task Force & UNESCO, 2024). For instance, the 2019 agreement set a timetable for contract teachers to enter the civil service and standardized pay scales. The agreements were implemented by joint government–union committees that monitor the rollout. The effectiveness here comes from formal negotiations; regular collective bargaining sessions are mandated by law, ensuring that teachers have a guaranteed voice on issues affecting them. This reduced unrest and raised the teaching profession's standing. Experts point out that Morocco's example shows that even in settings without a dedicated 'teacher council', strong union–government dialogue can meaningfully shape education.

3.2.8.2.3. Scotland: Co-constructing Curriculum and Policy. During the development of Scotland's Curriculum for Excellence (a sweeping curriculum reform), union representatives actively worked with government planners. Reports note that 'teacher unions in Scotland actively engage with planners on developing curricula and designing policies ... in a process of "co-construction"' (Teacher Task Force & UNESCO, 2024, p. 7). Practically, this meant the government held continuous consultations with the Educational Institute of Scotland (EIS) and the Scottish Secondary Teachers' Association (SSTA). Unions helped draft the professional standards for teachers and co-produced implementation guides. The result was a widely shared vision and a smoother rollout of the new curriculum (schools reported high teacher ownership). International observers highlight this model as enabling curriculum innovation while maintaining teacher morale.

4

DESIGNING SCHOOL ENVIRONMENTS FOR TEACHER WELL-BEING

Addressing teacher well-being at the school level requires a conceptual framework that moves beyond isolated wellness activities and acknowledges the full complexity of teachers' professional lives. A robust approach to teacher well-being must account for both the psychological dimensions of individual experience and the broader organizational conditions that shape those experiences. The PERMA model, developed by Seligman (2011), provides such a framework. It shifts the focus away from narrowly defined symptoms of stress or burnout and instead conceptualizes well-being as a multidimensional state of flourishing that can be cultivated through systemic support. At its core, the PERMA model identifies five interrelated domains that collectively define what it means to thrive: **P**ositive Emotion, **E**ngagement, **R**elationships, **M**eaning, and **A**chievement (Fig. 4).

The dimension of positive emotions reflects the affective tone of a teacher's workday, whether marked by appreciation, collegial joy, and moments of student connection, or dominated by fatigue, frustration, and emotional strain. Engagement speaks to whether teachers experience flow and intellectual stimulation in their instructional practice, or whether bureaucratic constraints and chronic overload sap their capacity to be fully present. Relationships refer to the social fabric of the school: the trust, empathy, and mutual respect that bind the staff together or, conversely, the isolation and conflict that can quietly erode morale. Meaning addresses the extent to which teachers feel that their work at school serves a greater purpose, aligns with their values, and contributes to something larger than themselves. Finally, achievement captures not just externally validated success but also a felt sense of efficacy, growth, and pride in one's professional contributions.

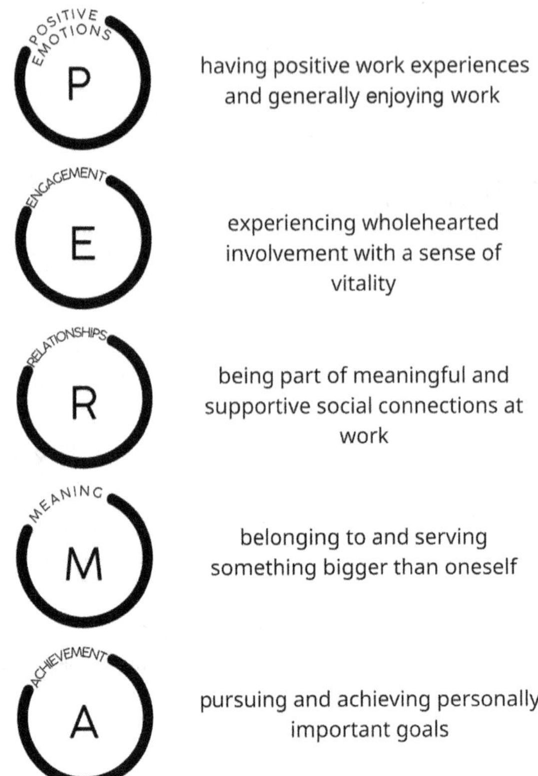

Fig. 4. PERMA Framework by Seligman (2011). Figure Created by the Author.

By articulating these five domains, PERMA allows school leaders and educators to take a more precise and systemic view of teacher well-being. It prompts questions that go beyond general satisfaction, such as: Are we intentionally designing opportunities for teachers to experience joy, engagement, and meaning in their daily work? Do our structures and norms support authentic collaboration and recognition? Are we cultivating a culture of shared purpose and professional growth?

Critically, the PERMA model emphasizes that well-being is not just an individual trait but a relational and organizational phenomenon. It is shaped by daily interactions, leadership behaviours, team dynamics, and institutional values. For school leaders seeking to support their staff meaningfully, PERMA offers more than a checklist. It provides a lens for understanding how individual well-being is intertwined with the school's norms, energy, and collective ethos, showing how a positive culture reinforces teachers' personal flourishing and creates a dynamic feedback loop in which individual and collective well-being are inseparable.

The following subsections present evidence of actions that school leaders can take to support teacher well-being. The measures are organized according to the PERMA framework, allowing leaders to explore strategies across different dimensions while considering how individual experiences and collective cultures interact to foster a resilient and thriving school environment. The following suggestions are grounded in PERMA theory and current research findings. If certain aspects appear to be missing, it may be due to a lack of empirical investigation or inconclusive evidence regarding their effectiveness.

4.1. FOSTER POSITIVE EMOTIONS AT SCHOOL

4.1.1. Psychological Safety

To be able to experience and enjoy positive emotions, teachers must have a firm psychological foundation, often referred to as psychological safety: a shared belief that the workplace is safe for interpersonal risk taking without fear of negative consequences. This sense of security is essential for fostering positive outcomes across various settings. Generally, when employees feel safe, they perform tasks more effectively, share knowledge openly, and go beyond their formal roles, creating a more dynamic and collaborative environment. In knowledge-driven contexts, psychological safety fuels creativity, vitality, and active engagement in learning behaviours. Additionally, meeting fundamental needs for connection and competence helps reduce fear, anxiety, and stress, thereby supporting mental health and strengthening commitment, especially among immigrant and minority groups. In high-pressure environments like child support, psychological safety encourages individuals to report suspicions despite fears of retaliation, promoting transparency and improvement. Its impact is further enhanced when employees feel confident in their expertise and authentic in their identities, underscoring the vital role of psychological safety in shaping inclusive, resilient workplaces.

In the teaching profession, psychological safety is closely linked to improved well-being and job satisfaction. When leaders and school communities foster a trusting, inclusive, and autonomy-supportive environment, teachers experience lower burnout, stronger commitment, and greater satisfaction with their work. Research from urban schools in the United States and Australian educational settings demonstrates that a clear psychosocial safety climate helps buffer the negative effects of high job demands. Interventions focused on supportive leadership, like training leaders to listen actively and fostering a sense of belonging within groups, have proven effective in enhancing psychological safety. Across diverse cultural and school contexts, it is clear that both organizational support and individual resources are critical for creating environments that are psychologically safe.

Literature reviewed: Belyaeva & Belyaeva, 2020; Carmeli et al., 2008; Carmeli et al., 2010; Collie et al., 2016; Derickson et al., 2015; Dreer-Goethe, 2025c; Ford et al., 2019; Gardner & Prasad, 2022; Garrick et al., 2014; Gerlach & Gockel, 2017; Itzchakov et al., 2022; Kamboj & Garg, 2021; Kark & Carmeli, 2008; Y. Liu & Keller, 2021; Mat Zin et al., 2023; Roffey, 2012; Siemsen et al., 2009; B. Singh et al., 2013; Sohail et al., 2023; Ulusoy et al., 2016.

4.1.1.1. Measure

Establish and sustain a psychologically safe school environment.

4.1.1.1.1. 3 Key Components

- **Learn how safe staff truly feel and act on it**

  Introduce feedback systems for evaluation, where teachers can anonymously reflect on how safe, heard, and respected they feel under their current leadership and within their school community. Use results to guide leadership development goals.

- **Establish a zero-tolerance policy for mobbing and microaggressions**

  Create and enforce clear, confidential procedures for reporting interpersonal harm such as mobbing, passive-aggressive behaviour, and microaggressions. Appoint a designated ombudsperson or psychological safety liaison (not necessarily an administrator) who can mediate early and escalate when necessary.

- **Make leadership behaviour visible and accountable**

  School leaders must publicly model the principles of psychological safety, like admitting their own mistakes, inviting dissenting views, and praising risk taking in teaching practice.

For Measure Dashboard, see Table 11.

Table 11. Measure Dashboard for Psychological Safety.

Dimension	Rating	Description
Impact	●●● **High**	Strong potential to transform teacher well-being. Addresses key drivers and has a broad, lasting impact
Quality of Evidence	●●● **High**	Strong, consistent evidence from rigorous research (e.g. meta-analyses, randomized controlled trials, longitudinal studies). Widely accepted in the field
Context Dependency	●○○ **Low**	Works effectively across most educational settings with minimal or no adaptation; broadly transferable
Sustainability	●●○ **Moderate**	Some integration into structures or culture, but still somewhat dependent on leadership or budget
Teacher Voice	●●○ **Moderate**	Some consultation with teachers, but limited decision-making power
Implementation Feasibility	●●○ **Moderate**	Requires some planning, adjustment, or collaboration. Feasible with committed leadership and moderate resource input

4.1.1.2. Good-Practice Example

4.1.1.2.1. United States: Anonymous Staff Climate Survey for Assessing Psychological Safety In the United States, school leaders can foster trust and psychological safety by implementing structured, anonymous staff climate surveys designed to surface honest feedback about leadership and school culture. Cult of Pedagogy offers a practical model in which educators are invited to reflect on their leadership strengths, identify growth areas, and suggest meaningful changes (Gonzalez, 2019). The survey includes both scaled questions (e.g. 'I feel comfortable approaching school leadership') and open-ended prompts (e.g. 'What is one thing you wish leadership understood better?'). Leaders are encouraged to review patterns in the responses without attempting to identify individuals, maintaining anonymity and preserving trust. This approach emphasizes transparency, reflection, and shared responsibility for school improvement – positioning feedback not as critique but as a tool for professional growth and relational repair.

4.1.2. Positive Work Experiences

Positive work experiences, like successfully guiding a student through a tricky problem and receiving a genuine 'well done' from a principal after a busy week, are essential contributors to teacher well-being and long-term engagement. Research shows that these experiences elevate positive emotions, increase job satisfaction, and buffer against the daily demands of emotional regulation. When teachers feel a sense of competence in their work, they report higher vitality, stronger motivation, and better mental health. A wide range of studies, spanning short-term interventions to long-term observational research, demonstrates that when positive experiences are cultivated intentionally, they create lasting improvements in emotional, cognitive, and physical well-being. One mechanism is the accumulation of positive events. When teachers repeatedly encounter moments of connection, success, or affirmation, these moments begin to build upon each other. This continuous exposure can create a buffer against stress and support sustained professional engagement.

Another reinforcing process is the development of positive spirals. When teachers reflect on positive experiences or discuss them with others, the emotional impact is strengthened, encouraging repetition and growth. Similarly, savouring can help extend the benefits of positive experiences. When educators take time to acknowledge and revisit meaningful moments, for example, through journaling, end-of-day reflections, or informal conversations with peers, they can amplify the emotional value of those moments. This reinforces well-being and improves memory and attention to future positives. Also, social sharing plays a vital role. When teachers talk about positive experiences with colleagues, whether in brief hallway conversations or more structured team meetings, they can elevate the experience.

Importantly, the positive impact of these experiences often extends beyond the workplace. Teachers who feel recognized, purposeful, and connected in school settings tend to carry those emotions into their personal lives. This phenomenon, known as cross-domain enrichment, can result in improved mood, better relationships at home, and greater overall life satisfaction.

While individual practices play a crucial role, research consistently shows that supportive organizational conditions are essential for sustaining positive experiences. Studies show that leadership that models savouring, builds optimism, and creates opportunities for reflection and growth is fundamental. When school environments prioritize emotional well-being, teachers are more likely to flourish.

Literature reviewed: Amabile et al., 2005; Arnold et al., 2007; Binnewies et al., 2009; Bono et al., 2013; Costantini & Sartori, 2018; Daniel & Sonnentag, 2014; Dimotakis et al., 2010; Feng & Han, 2023; K. E. Fox et al., 2021; Haworth et al., 1997; Hoobler et al., 2010; Ilies et al., 2024; Ilies et al., 2016; Malinowski & Lim, 2015; Ouweneel et al., 2013; Rivkin et al., 2018; Staw et al., 1994; Watkins et al., 2022; Weigelt et al., 2021.

4.1.2.1. Measure

Ensure that teachers regularly encounter and reflect on meaningful, affirming, and emotionally rewarding experiences.

4.1.2.1.1. 3 Key Components

- **Guarantee positive work experiences where you can**

  Because lessons can be unpredictable in how they feel for teachers, school leaders should create regular, simple moments that help teachers feel connected, appreciated, and uplifted.

- **Model and support emotional awareness practices**

  Train yourself to model savouring and optimism, openly sharing your own positive reflections on positive experiences as a leader.

- **Create structured moments for reflection and sharing**

  Establish regular opportunities, where teachers can revisit and savour positive moments. Encourage peer sharing during briefings or planning sessions to amplify and sustain the emotional benefits of positive experiences.

For Measure Dashboard, see Table 12.

Table 12. Measure Dashboard for Positive Work Experiences.

Dimension	Rating	Description
Impact	●●● **High**	Strong potential to transform teacher well-being. Addresses key drivers and has a broad, lasting impact
Quality of Evidence	●●● **High**	Strong, consistent evidence from rigorous research (e.g. meta-analyses, randomized controlled trials, longitudinal studies). Widely accepted in the field
Context Dependency	●○○ **Low**	Works effectively across most educational settings with minimal or no adaptation; broadly transferable
Sustainability	●●○ **Moderate**	Some integration into structures or culture, but still somewhat dependent on leadership or budget
Teacher Voice	●●● **High**	Teachers co-design, adapt, and lead the initiative; their professional knowledge is central
Implementation Feasibility	●●○ **Moderate**	Requires some planning, adjustment, or collaboration. Feasible with committed leadership and moderate resource input

4.1.2.2. Good-Practice Examples

4.1.2.2.1. England: A Systemic Approach to Staff Well-Being At Selly Park Girls' School in Birmingham, the commitment to teacher well-being is not an occasional initiative but a carefully embedded part of the school's organizational culture (Times Educational Supplement [TES], 2025). Awarded the TES Staff Wellbeing School of the Year 2025, the school has developed an integrated system that tackles the root causes of stress, from workload management to leadership openness. Policies such as streamlined marking practices, staggered parent evenings, and flexible work-from-home arrangements ensure that teachers experience a manageable balance between professional responsibilities and personal time. Alongside this, redesigned staff spaces, a mindfulness room, and opportunities for social connection provide an environment where teachers feel valued and supported. Importantly, the leadership models transparency and maintains an open-door culture, encouraging staff to voice concerns early and collaboratively find solutions. The result is an atmosphere where positive professional experiences, such as being recognized for good work, feeling trusted, and maintaining healthy boundaries, are consistently reinforced. Staff surveys show near-universal agreement that well-being is a school priority, and teacher turnover remains exceptionally low. This example demonstrates how a coherent, systemic approach can transform everyday work experiences for teachers into sustainable sources of motivation, belonging, and professional pride.

4.1.2.2.2. India: Teacher Well-Being Through Structured Collaboration Iqbalia International School was recognized by Adhvaith Foundation in 2017 for its teacher-centred culture. Every Saturday, teachers gather in a 'circle time' session where each person shares a meaningful positive experience from the week (Saleem, 2024). Initially, staff found it hard to focus on good moments, but over time, these weekly reflections became a powerful ritual. Teachers reported a greater awareness of positive moments, stronger peer bonds, and a heightened sense of emotional energy and pride in their work. This practice of structured reflection and savouring mirrors research findings that show that routinely noticing and socially sharing successes reinforces positivity spirals and improves teacher well-being—making everyday work emotionally rewarding and connective rather than transactional.

4.1.3. Culture of Appreciation

A school culture of appreciation that includes genuine recognition, supportive behaviour, and clear, respectful communication is consistently associated with improved teacher well-being. Leadership appreciation that includes genuine recognition, supportive behaviour, and clear, respectful communication is linked to enhanced teacher well-being and job satisfaction. Recent research highlights that when school leaders express sincere praise, gratitude, and affirmation, teachers feel more valued and connected, fostering greater engagement and psychological safety. This appreciation nurtures a positive emotional climate, strengthening relational trust and encouraging openness within the school community. Supportive leadership behaviours, such as mentoring, constructive feedback, and ongoing, meaningful dialogue, help reduce stress and promote professional growth. Importantly, recent findings from a large study of German teachers reveal that appreciation from school leaders has the strongest and most consistent impact on all aspects of teacher well-being, including job satisfaction, emotional exhaustion, and intentions to quit. Appreciation from students and colleagues also plays a significant role, while recognition from more distant sources such as policymakers and society has less direct influence. These insights underscore that leadership appreciation is most effective when embedded within a culture of trust and shared values, reinforcing a sense of belonging and professional identity. Such environments mitigate burnout and empower teachers to thrive, making appreciation a vital, ongoing practice for sustaining emotionally healthy, high-performing schools.

Literature reviewed: Baggett et al., 2016; Cvenkel, 2018; Dreer-Goethe, 2025b; Gregersen et al., 2014; Kelloway, Turner, et al., 2012; Kelloway, Weigand, et al., 2012; Stocker et al., 2014; Stocker et al., 2019; Vincent-Höper et al., 2017; Westover, 2025; Winkler et al., 2014.

4.1.3.1. Measure

Build a culture of genuine appreciation and supportive communication.

4.1.3.1.1. 3 Key Components

- **Practice regular, sincere recognition**

  School leaders should consistently express authentic praise, gratitude, and affirmation tailored to individual teacher contributions.

- **Encourage multisource appreciation**

  Promote a culture where appreciation flows not only from leadership but also among colleagues and students.

- **Ensure that appreciation includes you as a leader**

  Put structures in place that allow you to receive genuine appreciation and constructive feedback as well. This helps maintain your well-being while energizing your continued practice of appreciation.

For Measure Dashboard, see Table 13.

4.1.3.2. Good-Practice Example

4.1.3.2.1. United States: Building School Culture with Gratitude Through GiveThx Leadership in Public Schools in Oakland, California, implemented a research-informed, inclusive approach to embed gratitude into everyday school life by combining a curriculum with a digital tool to reinforce specific positive behaviours among students and staff (Fauteux, 2018). Originally using informal verbal shout-outs, they moved to an accessible system called GiveThx (https://www.givethx.org), a web app that lets students and teachers anonymously send digital thank-you notes to each other after demonstrating key school values. Crucially, the approach is paired with a structured gratitude curriculum, co-designed with a psychology expert, that explicitly teaches behaviours linked to emotional well-being and belonging. Early findings showed increased student life and friendship satisfaction, reduced stress and anxiety, and enhanced visibility of positive actions.

Table 13. Measure Dashboard for Culture of Appreciation.

Dimension	**Rating**	**Description**
Impact	●●● **High**	Strong potential to transform teacher well-being. Addresses key drivers and has a broad, lasting impact
Quality of Evidence	●●● **High**	Strong, consistent evidence from rigorous research (e.g. meta-analyses, randomized controlled trials, longitudinal studies). Widely accepted in the field
Context Dependency	●○○ **Low**	Works effectively across most educational settings with minimal or no adaptation; broadly transferable
Sustainability	●●○ **Moderate**	Some integration into structures or culture, but still somewhat dependent on leadership or budget
Teacher Voice	●●● **High**	Teachers co-design, adapt, and lead the initiative; their professional knowledge is central
Implementation Feasibility	●●○ **Moderate**	Requires some planning, adjustment, or collaboration. Feasible with committed leadership and moderate resource input

4.2. PROMOTE TEACHER ENGAGEMENT

4.2.1. Teaching Autonomy

Teaching autonomy is central to teacher engagement and well-being. When teachers can make decisions about curriculum and instructional methods, they experience lower stress, stronger professional identity, and a greater sense of purpose. By contrast, excessive bureaucracy and rigid managerial controls undermine autonomy, contributing to disengagement and emotional exhaustion. Research consistently links autonomy to higher job satisfaction, motivation, and retention. Leadership that fosters autonomy and cultivates a supportive school culture further strengthens these outcomes, while restrictive practices increase turnover intentions. Ultimately, promoting autonomy through organizational policies and leadership is key to enhancing teacher well-being and sustaining engagement.

> Literature reviewed: Brady & Wilson, 2020; Collie, 2023; Fradkin-Hayslip, 2021; Jerrim et al., 2023; Pan et al., 2023; Pearson & Moomaw, 2005; Perry et al., 2015; Skaalvik & Skaalvik, 2014; Skinner et al., 2019.

4.2.1.1. Measure

Foster teaching autonomy by empowering decisions, easing constraints, and leading supportively.

4.2.1.1.1. 3 Key Components

- **Empower curriculum-level decision-making**

  Give teachers the freedom to shape lesson plans, select materials, and adapt instruction to meet student needs within a broad, shared framework to enhance ownership and reduce stress.

- **Reduce unnecessary constraints**

  Audit and revise routines, reporting tasks, and compliance processes to eliminate bureaucratic burdens that limit teachers' professional judgement and autonomy.

- **Be an autonomy-supportive leader**

  Adopt coaching and trust-based approaches that validate teachers' expertise, invite input into school priorities, and foster a culture of shared professionalism.

For Measure Dashboard, see Table 14.

4.2.1.2. Good-Practice Example

4.2.1.2.1. United States: Empowering Teachers Through Autonomy The A.D. Henderson School in Boca Raton, Florida, is consistently ranked among the state's top-performing public schools and has been highlighted in recent reports for its distinctive commitment to teacher autonomy (Spencer, 2024). Rather than imposing scripted curricula or rigid instructional pacing, the school empowers educators to design and lead their own classroom experiences, often involving hands-on projects and interdisciplinary learning. Teachers are trusted as professionals and encouraged to innovate, while leadership deliberately focuses on support rather than oversight. This autonomy is embedded in a school culture that prioritizes mutual respect, professional trust, and long-term commitment. Staff report high levels of job satisfaction and engagement, with many remaining at the school for decades. According to coverage, this autonomy-focused model not only strengthens teacher well-being but also contributes to a consistently positive school climate and sustained academic excellence.

Table 14. Measure Dashboard for Autonomy.

Dimension	Rating	Description
Impact	●●● **High**	Strong potential to transform teacher well-being. Addresses key drivers and has a broad, lasting impact
Quality of Evidence	●●● **High**	Strong, consistent evidence from rigorous research (e.g. meta-analyses, randomized controlled trials, longitudinal studies). Widely accepted in the field
Context Dependency	●○○ **Low**	Works effectively across most educational settings with minimal or no adaptation; broadly transferable
Sustainability	●●○ **Moderate**	Some integration into structures or culture, but still somewhat dependent on leadership or budget
Teacher Voice	●●● **High**	Teachers co-design, adapt, and lead the initiative; their professional knowledge is central
Implementation Feasibility	●●○ **Moderate**	Requires some planning, adjustment, or collaboration. Feasible with committed leadership and moderate resource input

4.2.2. Harmonious Passion

Harmonious passion, when teachers feel a genuine, self-driven connection to their work, has been linked to greater job satisfaction and lower levels of burnout. Teachers who experience this kind of passion often report feeling more effective, emotionally balanced, and energized in the classroom. They are more likely to engage in creative and meaningful teaching practices because their motivation comes from within, rather than from pressure or obligation. On the other hand, obsessive passion, which feels more like a compulsion, tends to be associated with emotional exhaustion and detachment. What makes the difference is how schools support teachers; when autonomy, emotional support, and opportunities for meaningful engagement are present, passion becomes a source of strength rather than stress. These findings point to the importance of creating school environments where teachers can connect with their work in healthy, fulfilling ways.

Literature reviewed: Burić & Moè, 2020; Carbonneau et al., 2008; Castillo et al., 2017; Crosswell & Elliott, 2004; Day & Kington, 2008; Fernet et al., 2014; Fogelgarn & Burns, 2020; Kasprzak & Mudło-Głagolska, 2022; Kun & Gadanecz, 2019; Önder, 2019; Schiefele et al., 2013; Yin et al., 2018.

4.2.2.1. Measure

Create an atmosphere where teachers feel encouraged to bring their personal interests into their work.

4.2.2.1.1. 3 Key Components

- **Cultivate a culture of experimentation and risk-taking**

  Encourage teachers to try new teaching methods and ideas in their classrooms. Create safe spaces, like a 'failure-friendly forum' where teachers can openly share what they have learnt from challenges.

- **Actively recognize and share teacher expertise**

  Establish regular opportunities for staff to present their work and interests. Promote widespread participation and frame these contributions as valuable leadership in practice.

- **Encourage subject passion and professional learning**

  Encourage teachers to pursue in-depth study or enrichment in the subjects they love. Support side passion projects with small grants or resources to help teachers explore new approaches without the fear of failure.

For Measure Dashboard, see Table 15.

4.2.2.2. Good-Practice Examples

4.2.2.2.1. Canada: Building Teacher Leadership Through Passion Projects At Milton District High School in Ontario, Canada, school leadership launched a teacher-driven passion projects initiative as part of a broader effort to shift school culture and leadership (Cronin, 2018). Special education resource teachers were invited to identify a topic of professional or personal interest and were given dedicated time and coverage to work on their projects during the school day. Topics ranged from exploring staff wellness and creating department websites to rethinking pedagogical supports for students.

Leadership actively supported this process by adjusting schedules. The lead educator even covered classes herself to ensure teachers had the time to engage meaningfully. A key element of the project was its informality – staff met over coffee, kept connected through social media, and were encouraged to reflect publicly and informally. As a result, teachers reported renewed energy, professional growth, and deeper relationships.

Table 15. Measure Dashboard 15 for Harmonious Passion.

Dimension	Rating	Description
Impact	●●● **High**	Strong potential to transform teacher well-being. Addresses key drivers and has a broad, lasting impact
Quality of Evidence	●●○ **Moderate**	Some research support, possibly from case studies or correlational data. Promising but not conclusive
Context Dependency	●○○ **Low**	Works effectively across most educational settings with minimal or no adaptation; broadly transferable
Sustainability	●●○ **Moderate**	Some integration into structures or culture, but still somewhat dependent on leadership or budget
Teacher Voice	●●● **High**	Teachers co-design, adapt, and lead the initiative; their professional knowledge is central
Implementation Feasibility	●●○ **Moderate**	Requires some planning, adjustment, or collaboration. Feasible with committed leadership and moderate resource input

4.2.2.2.2. England: Teacher-Led Spotlights Week Empowering Staff and Elevating Voice

In Essex, England, a network of primary and secondary schools implemented Spotlights Week, a school-led initiative in which teachers design and lead professional development sessions based on their personal expertise and passions (Essex Research School, 2025). Topics include everything from forest school pedagogy and trauma-informed teaching to music education and team leadership. These sessions are delivered by teachers for teachers, creating a culture of shared learning, trust, and empowerment across schools. Leaders report that participation boosts teacher confidence, professional identity, and morale (Essex Research School, 2025). Importantly, it is not limited to formal roles. Any teacher with something to share is invited to present, reinforcing the idea that all educators bring value and leadership potential. Spotlights Week has become a scalable, low-cost model for recognizing and supporting passion-driven practices in everyday school development.

4.2.3. Flow

Flow – a state in which action and awareness blend seamlessly under conditions of balanced challenge and skill – is increasingly recognized as a meaningful contributor to teacher well-being. Across various studies, teachers who experience flow describe heightened enjoyment, a strong sense of control, and increased clarity around instructional goals. Many report moments of complete immersion in teaching, marked by a sense of automaticity and losing track of time. These experiences often coincide with reduced feelings of burnout and greater work engagement. Flow is influenced by multiple factors, including subject matter interest, intrinsic motivation, supportive leadership, design of learning spaces, and positive classroom dynamics. While definitions and measurement approaches differ, the overall pattern is consistent – when teachers are able to engage deeply and purposefully in their teaching, they are more likely to feel emotionally fulfilled, professionally optimistic, and satisfied in their roles.

> Literature reviewed: Basom & Frase, 2004; Bassi & Fave, 2012; Beard & Hoy, 2010; Schiefele et al., 2013; Tardy, 2004; Zausmer et al., 2024; Zilka et al., 2023.

4.2.3.1. Measure

Foster conditions that enable teachers to experience flow in their daily work.

4.2.3.1.1. 3 Key Components

- **Make flow a shared topic of professional reflection**

  Integrate the concept of flow into staff meetings, professional development, and teacher evaluations as a lens for understanding engagement. Encourage teachers to reflect on when they feel most absorbed and energized in their work and what conditions support that.

- **Support teachers in shaping their own teaching spaces**

  Empower teachers to co-design their classrooms to reflect their teaching style, subject needs, and the types of engagement they value. Whether through flexible furniture, wall displays, or zones for different activities, allowing teachers to personalize their space strengthens their sense of ownership and flow.

- **Create opportunities for deep work**

  Reorganize schedules to allow longer, uninterrupted blocks of teaching or planning time. Protecting this space from meetings or administrative demands enables deeper cognitive engagement.

For Measure Dashboard, see Table 16.

4.2.3.2. Good-Practice Example

4.2.3.2.1. Portugal: Co-designed Classrooms Foster Flow-Friendly Teaching Environments The TEL@FTELab (Technology Enhanced Learning @ Future Teacher Education Lab) project (Pedro et al., 2017), led by the University of

Table 16. Measure Dashboard for Flow.

Dimension	Rating	Description
Impact	●●○ **Moderate**	Has a noticeable effect for some contexts or groups. Contributes meaningfully but not comprehensively
Quality of Evidence	●●○ **Moderate**	Some research support, possibly from case studies or correlational data. Promising but not conclusive
Context Dependency	●○○ **Low**	Works effectively across most educational settings with minimal or no adaptation; broadly transferable
Sustainability	●●○ **Moderate**	Some integration into structures or culture, but still somewhat dependent on leadership or budget
Teacher Voice	●●● **High**	Teachers co-design, adapt, and lead the initiative; their professional knowledge is central
Implementation Feasibility	●●○ **Moderate**	Requires some planning, adjustment, or collaboration. Feasible with committed leadership and moderate resource input

Lisbon, offers a concrete example of how co-designed learning environments can support conditions that promote teacher flow. Through a participatory design process, in-service teachers, future teachers, students, architects, and designers collaboratively envisioned and prototyped the 'classroom of the future'. Using tools like mock-ups, 3D modelling, and virtual reality, participants worked in small groups to design flexible, reconfigurable classroom layouts that prioritize comfort, collaboration, autonomy, and embedded technology. Teachers emphasized the need for spaces that support diversified, student-centred pedagogies while also enabling greater teacher agency in how space is used, highlighting key flow enablers like clarity, autonomy, and optimal challenge. Findings showed strong consensus among stakeholders that future classrooms must accommodate different modes of teaching and learning simultaneously through multipurpose zones, movable furniture, ample natural light, and reliable wireless connectivity. These design elements directly contribute to a teaching environment conducive to flow by minimizing environmental friction, promoting focus, and fostering intrinsic motivation.

4.2.4. Professional Development

When professional development is sustained, responsive, and tailored to individual needs, it cultivates professional engagement and a stronger sense of efficacy. Teachers who participate in well-designed programmes often describe a shift from narrowly defined performance goals to broader, value-driven professional identities. In some cases, the lack of alignment between professional development content and teacher priorities has led to resistance, underscoring the importance of relevance and respect for educators' contexts.

Across a wide range of studies, the most impactful professional development initiatives are those that integrate reflection, mentorship, and holistic well-being. These programmes go beyond technical skill building to support teachers' mental, emotional, and professional growth, ultimately helping to retain motivated educators and foster healthier school communities.

Professional development programmes that prioritize mindfulness, social–emotional learning, and individualized support have shown consistent links to enhanced teacher well-being. Evidence from diverse educational contexts demonstrates that such programmes can help reduce stress, build emotional resilience, and foster a renewed sense of purpose in teaching. Programmes that integrate mindfulness practices and coaching have led to noticeable improvements in emotion regulation and psychological balance, contributing to teachers' sense of joy and confidence in their roles. Creative and arts-based approaches have also been associated with higher levels of resilience and reduced signs of secondary stress.

Collectively, these findings suggest that professional development formats combining collaboration, resource investment, and strong school support contribute to enhanced teacher engagement and well-being, as evidenced by multiple research designs and contextual settings.

> Literature reviewed: AlHussaini et al., 2024; Anderson et al., 2022; Belmonte et al., 2022; Cann et al., 2024; Carpenter et al., 2023; Compen et al., 2020; Dreer et al., 2017; Eun & Heining-Boynton, 2007; Even-Zahav et al., 2022; Fowler et al., 2022; Y. He & Bagwell, 2021; Ingvarson et al., 2005; Jennings et al., 2017; Ji, 2021, 2025; Kelly et al., 2022; King, 2012; Mouza, 2009; Robinette, 2024; Vicuña Delos Reyes, 2024; Walter et al., 2023; X. Wang & Chen, 2022.

4.2.4.1. Measure

Empower teaching staff through sustained, responsive professional development that supports their well-being and professional purpose.

4.2.4.1.1. 3 Key Components

- **Embed well-being into professional development planning**

  Ensure that professional development offerings explicitly address teacher well-being. This includes integrating practices like mindfulness, creative expression, and social–emotional learning into professional development schedules as central elements that acknowledge the emotional demands of teaching.

- **Co-design professional development with teachers**

  Involve teachers in shaping professional development priorities instead of prescribing top-down content. By conducting regular needs assessments, hosting collaborative planning sessions, and adapting content to different career stages and roles, leaders show respect for teacher autonomy and increase the relevance and uptake of training opportunities.

- **Foster ongoing support networks**

  To make learning sustainable, facilitate mentorship programmes, encourage peer coaching, and create time for reflective dialogue among staff. These structures build a culture of continuous learning in which teachers feel supported, valued, and professionally engaged.

For Measure Dashboard, see Table 17.

Table 17. Measure Dashboard for Professional Development.

Dimension	Rating	Description
Impact	●●● **High**	Strong potential to transform teacher well-being. Addresses key drivers and has a broad, lasting impact
Quality of Evidence	●●● **High**	Strong, consistent evidence from rigorous research (e.g. meta-analyses, randomized controlled trials, longitudinal studies). Widely accepted in the field
Context Dependency	●○○ **Low**	Works effectively across most educational settings with minimal or no adaptation; broadly transferable
Sustainability	●○○ **Low**	Requires ongoing external input or funding; unlikely to persist without constant support
Teacher Voice	●●● **High**	Teachers co-design, adapt, and lead the initiative; their professional knowledge is central
Implementation Feasibility	●●○ **Moderate**	Requires some planning, adjustment, or collaboration. Feasible with committed leadership and moderate resource input

4.2.4.2. Good-Practice Example

4.2.4.2.1. Aotearoa New Zealand: MARKERS Well-being Program for Educators The MARKERS Wellbeing Program for Educators (Cann et al., 2024) stands out as a good-practice example of professional development that meaningfully enhances teacher well-being through a deeply contextual, multilayered approach. Rather than applying a generic framework, the programme was designed using a theory-of-change model tailored to the specific needs and culture of the participating school. It addressed teacher well-being across three interconnected levels. At the individual level, teachers engaged in self-care workshops, mindfulness training, and resilience-building exercises that helped them develop personal coping strategies. At the relational level, the programme facilitated peer sessions, reflective group discussions, and collaborative activities to strengthen collegial support and rebuild trust among staff. Critically, the contextual level involved active participation from school leadership, who worked to integrate well-being priorities into the school's everyday practices and policies.

What makes this programme particularly compelling is its adaptability. Rather than being rigid, it was continuously shaped by ongoing reflection and feedback from teachers and leaders, allowing the structure, delivery, and content to evolve in real time. Teachers reported significant improvements in their overall well-being, noting greater emotional balance, stronger resilience, and a renewed sense of job satisfaction. The school climate itself shifted, with staff describing more positive daily interactions and a stronger sense of professional community. Because leadership was involved throughout the process as co-participants, the initiative was seen not as a one-off intervention but as a shared commitment to a healthier, more sustainable school culture.

4.3. BUILD SUPPORTIVE PROFESSIONAL RELATIONSHIPS

4.3.1. Trust

Trust in leaders, colleagues, and the broader organization plays a pivotal role in shaping well-being across both teaching and general workplace settings. In broader employee contexts, trust in leadership similarly correlates with higher job satisfaction and reduced stress. For teachers, trust in principals, peers, and even students is consistently linked to greater job satisfaction, deeper engagement, and improved mental health, including reduced burnout and emotional exhaustion. In contrast, the absence of trust can be costly. Teachers who lack trust in their school leadership report significantly higher levels of burnout. Importantly, trust not only has a direct impact; it also serves as a powerful mediator and moderator. It amplifies the positive effects of transformational leadership, mitigates the strain of heavy workloads, and shapes how human resource practices influence well-being. These dynamics are further influenced by contextual factors such as available resources, organizational climate, and situational challenges, like the shift to virtual teaching during the COVID-19 pandemic, highlighting trust as both a stabilizing and enabling force in complex professional environments.

> Literature reviewed: Alfes et al., 2012; Ceyanes & Slater, 2005; Huang et al., 2019; Kelloway, Turner, et al., 2012; Labarthe-Carrara et al., 2024; J. Liu et al., 2010; Tsuyuguchi, 2023; Van Maele & Van Houtte, 2015; Yin et al., 2016.

4.3.1.1. Measure

Build and sustain trust through transparent, supportive, and consistent leadership practices.

4.3.1.1.1. 3 Key Components

- **Communicate transparently and follow through on commitments**

  Leaders should share decisions, priorities, and changes openly, especially when the news is difficult. Trust is built when communication is honest and expectations are clear. Just as importantly, leaders must reliably follow through on promises, timelines, and agreed-upon support, showing teachers that their words are backed by action.

- **Create possibilities for honest dialogue**

  Establish means for teachers to voice concerns, suggest improvements, or raise emotional or workload-related challenges without fear of reprisal. Ensure that feedback loops are closed by transparently reporting what is heard and what actions will follow.

- **Model humility**

  Trust deepens when leaders acknowledge their own limitations, admit mistakes, and invite critical feedback from staff. This signals that it is safe to be human, take risks, and speak up.

For Measure Dashboard, see Table 18.

Table 18. Measure Dashboard for Trust.

Dimension	Rating	Description
Impact	●●● **High**	Strong potential to transform teacher well-being. Addresses key drivers and has a broad, lasting impact
Quality of Evidence	●●● **High**	Strong, consistent evidence from rigorous research (e.g. meta-analyses, randomized controlled trials, longitudinal studies). Widely accepted in the field
Context Dependency	●○○ **Low**	Works effectively across most educational settings with minimal or no adaptation; broadly transferable
Sustainability	●●○ **Moderate**	Some integration into structures or culture, but still somewhat dependent on leadership or budget
Teacher Voice	●●○ **Moderate**	Some consultation with teachers, but limited decision-making power
Implementation Feasibility	●●○ **Moderate**	Requires some planning, adjustment, or collaboration. Feasible with committed leadership and moderate resource input

4.3.1.2. Good-Practice Example

4.3.1.2.1. South Korea: Building Trust Through Shared Leadership In several South Korean high schools, principals have been rethinking leadership to build trust and collaboration with their staff. Instead of making decisions behind closed doors, these leaders create regular open forums where teachers help shape school goals, policies, and classroom initiatives. This approach, also known as participatory leadership, gives teachers a sense of ownership and reduces the traditional hierarchy between staff and leadership. What makes this work especially well in South Korea's context is the focus on respectful dialogue and collective problem-solving. Principals deliberately model humility by listening first, admitting when they do not have all the answers, and showing appreciation for staff ideas. Teachers, in turn, feel valued and safe to contribute honestly. Over time, this trust encourages staff to share challenges openly and experiment with new teaching practices without fear of criticism. Research on two South Korean high schools shows that principals who practise participatory and transformational leadership build strong trust between staff and leadership (Kang & Printy, 2009). These practices create safer, more collaborative environments where teachers feel valued and are motivated to innovate.

4.3.2. Social Support

Workplace social support plays a crucial role in enhancing employee well-being by reducing burnout, stress, depression, and anxiety while increasing job satisfaction and emotional resilience. Support from supervisors and organizational sources consistently shows the strongest positive effects, working through both direct emotional benefits and indirect mechanisms such as psychological empowerment and stress regulation. Positive professional outcomes often accompany higher levels of social support, and factors like personal well-being, self-efficacy, and social network structures help explain its impact. However, the quality, type, and context of support matter greatly. Support that is well-tailored to individual needs and specific stressors is most effective, while poorly matched support may have mixed or even adverse effects.

In educational settings, teachers report that social support reduces burnout, emotional exhaustion, and stress while enhancing job satisfaction, teaching effectiveness, and self-esteem. Support from colleagues, supervisors, and school leaders buffers against work overload and emotional exhaustion, promoting feelings of personal accomplishment and improving mental health. Perceived organizational support also strengthens work engagement and coping. These benefits are evident across diverse regions and educational levels, emphasizing the importance of tailored, high-quality support to sustain teacher well-being and effectiveness.

Literature reviewed: Brough & Pears, 2004; Brouwers et al., 2001; Chi et al., 2014; Ghasemi, 2022; Greenglass et al., 1997; Greenglass et al., 1996; Griffith et al., 1999; Kaihoi et al., 2022; Kinman et al., 2011; Moeller & Chung-Yan, 2013; Ransford et al., 2009; Ray & Miller, 1991; Russell et al., 1987; Sarros & Sarros, 1992; Schonfeld, 2001; Senarathna & Ranasinghe, 2024; Temam et al., 2019; X. Yu et al., 2024; Zinsser et al., 2016.

4.3.2.1. Measure

Cultivate a working culture of proactive, tailored social support.

4.3.2.1.1. 3 Key Components

- **Create micro-spaces and moments for spontaneous interaction**

  Design physical and digital spaces and deliberately protect unstructured time that makes social connections more likely. Examples include a well-placed staff coffee table or vending machine, a rotating 'appreciation wall' in the lounge, or a 'well-being board' in the staff room.

- **Map social support networks**

  Use surveys or short interviews to visualize social support flows. Identify whom teachers turn to for emotional or practical help and uncover bottlenecks or feelings of isolation.

- **Form adaptive support teams**

  Bring together small groups of teachers and leaders regularly to analyze support maps and co-design targeted actions such as buddy systems, resource shifts, or stress relief activities.

For Measure Dashboard, see Table 19.

Table 19. Measure Dashboard 19 for Social Support.

Dimension	Rating	Description
Impact	●●● **High**	Strong potential to transform teacher well-being. Addresses key drivers and has a broad, lasting impact
Quality of Evidence	●●● **High**	Strong, consistent evidence from rigorous research (e.g. meta-analyses, randomized controlled trials, longitudinal studies). Widely accepted in the field
Context Dependency	●●○ **Moderate**	Requires some adaptation but can function in several settings; effectiveness depends on moderately specific conditions (e.g. type of school)
Sustainability	●●○ **Moderate**	Some integration into structures or culture, but still somewhat dependent on leadership or budget
Teacher Voice	●●● **High**	Teachers co-design, adapt, and lead the initiative; their professional knowledge is central
Implementation Feasibility	●●○ **Moderate**	Requires some planning, adjustment, or collaboration. Feasible with committed leadership and moderate resource input

4.3.2.2. Good-Practice Example

4.3.2.2.1. United States: 'tap-in/tap-out' System as a Model for Workplace Social Support Fall-Hamilton Elementary in Nashville, Tennessee, has implemented a 'tap-in/tap-out' system that provides a structured yet flexible way for teachers to access immediate social and emotional support during the school day (Terada, 2023). When a teacher feels overwhelmed or needs a break, they can send a brief, explanation-free text message to a designated school number or support team. This support can be requested for any reason, whether due to emotional stress, behavioural challenges in the classroom, or simply needing a moment to self-regulate. Within minutes, two trained staff members respond. One staff member 'taps in' by entering the classroom and taking over instruction, ensuring students are supervised and learning continues uninterrupted. Meanwhile, the second staff member 'taps out' with the teacher, offering a check-in, emotional support, or simply providing time and space for the teacher to regroup, whether that's a few minutes in a quiet area, a walk, or a private conversation.

This system eliminates the pressure on teachers to justify their need for a break and reinforces the message that it is both acceptable and encouraged to seek help. By building this kind of responsive support into the school day, staff are better able to regulate themselves, avoid burnout, and return to their classrooms feeling more grounded and effective. The continued use of the tap-in/tap-out model, even after leadership transitions, highlights its value and sustainability as a good practice for tailored social support.

4.3.3. Student–Teacher Relationships

Positive student–teacher relationships are a powerful factor in sustaining teacher well-being. When teachers experience consistent, respectful, and emotionally supportive interactions with students, they are more likely to feel fulfilled in their roles, report higher job satisfaction, and show resilience against burnout. These relationships act as a buffer against the daily stresses of teaching, helping to reduce emotional exhaustion and feelings of depersonalization. Conversely, ongoing conflict or negative dynamics with students can drain teachers emotionally, heighten stress, and erode their sense of professional efficacy. Especially in challenging environments or crisis situations, the quality of student–teacher relationships can either ease or intensify the emotional toll of the work. This underscores the need for school cultures that foster mutual respect, empathy, and connection in the classroom.

> Literature reviewed: Corbin et al., 2019; Falk et al., 2022; Haldimann et al., 2023; Harding et al., 2019; Milatz et al., 2015; Poulou, 2020; Rafsanjani et al., 2019; Roffey, 2012; S. Yoon, 2002; Shen et al., 2015.

4.3.3.1. Measure

Support positive student–teacher relationships.

4.3.3.1.1. 3 Key Components

- **Champion a culture of relational teaching**

  Encourage and model a school-wide ethos where building positive relationships with students is seen as central to teaching. This can be reinforced through professional development, staff meetings, and recognition systems that celebrate relational excellence.

- **Train teachers in relational and emotional skills**

  Offer training on classroom management, de-escalation strategies, trauma-informed teaching, and emotional intelligence. These tools help teachers build positive relationships and manage difficult student behaviour.

- **Intervene supportively in chronic student–teacher conflict**

  When relationships between teachers and specific students become strained, step in supportively—not punitively. This might involve co-developing action plans, offering conflict mediation, or pairing teachers with behavioural specialists to analyze the situation and find constructive paths forward.

For Measure Dashboard, see Table 20.

4.3.3.2. Good-Practice Example

4.3.3.2.1. Nepal: Building Positive Relationships Through Relational Teaching in Rural Schools In the remote mountain communities of Nepal, the Himalayan Trust (REED Nepal) has transformed the emotional climate of classrooms through a teacher training programme that prioritizes human connection over discipline (Himalayan Trust UK, 2025). Where classrooms were once marked by fear and rigid control, they have become vibrant, child-centred learning spaces rooted in warmth, respect, and relational teaching. Teachers now greet every child by name with a smile, encourage participation, and replace punishment with praise. Simple daily gestures have built strong bonds of trust and mutual respect. Former 'stick corners' have been replaced with reading corners, handmade learning materials, and cooperative group activities that engage every student. These shifts have had profound effects. Headteachers and programme coordinators report that this relational approach has

Table 20. Measure Dashboard 20 for Student–Teacher Relationships.

Dimension	Rating	Description
Impact	●●● **High**	Strong potential to transform teacher well-being. Addresses key drivers and has a broad, lasting impact
Quality of Evidence	●●● **High**	Strong, consistent evidence from rigorous research (e.g. meta-analyses, randomized controlled trials, longitudinal studies). Widely accepted in the field
Context Dependency	●○○ **Low**	Works effectively across most educational settings with minimal or no adaptation; broadly transferable
Sustainability	●●○ **Moderate**	Some integration into structures or culture, but still somewhat dependent on leadership or budget
Teacher Voice	●●● **High**	Teachers co-design, adapt, and lead the initiative; their professional knowledge is central
Implementation Feasibility	●●○ **Moderate**	Requires some planning, adjustment, or collaboration. Feasible with committed leadership and moderate resource input

transformed not only student engagement but also teacher well-being. Teachers feel more connected to their students, more fulfilled in their roles, and more resilient in the face of challenges. The ripple effects extend beyond the classroom, strengthening relationships with parents and the wider community and creating a school culture grounded in care, participation, and joy.

4.3.4. Playfulness

Emerging research suggests that playfulness is connected with warmer classroom relationships and a more positive school culture. Research from Denmark showed that playful participatory methods fostered positive shifts in teacher identity and promoted a willingness to experiment within classroom settings. However, its association with self-efficacy appears to depend on the cultural and institutional setting. In Indonesia, a study of early childhood teachers reported a significant negative correlation between playfulness and self-efficacy. In Turkey, pressures from academic and parental expectations were linked to reduced playful engagement.

> Literature reviewed: Baker & Ryan, 2021; Canaslan-Akyar & Sevimli-Celik, 2021; Dierenfeld, 2024; Farley et al., 2021; Winy Nila, 2024.

4.3.4.1. Measure

Foster a culture of playfulness.

4.3.4.1.1. 3 Key Components

- **Encourage playful, participatory teaching methods**

  Support teachers in integrating playful approaches in their classrooms to build warmer student–teacher relationships and promote creativity and experimentation in teaching.

- **Create supportive spaces for teacher experimentation**

  Establish forums or peer groups where teachers can share playful practices, reflect on their experiences, and adapt methods without fear of judgement or pressure, fostering a positive school culture.

- **Provide culturally responsive professional development**

  Offer training that recognizes cultural and institutional contexts, helping teachers balance playfulness with academic expectations and build confidence in their unique environments.

For Measure Dashboard, see Table 21.

4.3.4.2. Good-Practice Example

4.3.4.2.1. Denmark: Playful Participatory Research Transforms Teacher Learning At the International School of Billund in Denmark, a powerful example of teacher-led professional development emerged through playful participatory research, a collaboration with Project Zero at Harvard (Baker & Ryan, 2021). Rooted in the school's philosophy of learning through play, the project engaged teachers as co-researchers in small study groups, where they explored classroom documentation, posed their own questions, and reflected in intentionally playful environments. Supported by school leadership with dedicated time and resources, the method fostered professional growth, a playful mindset, and a stronger sense of community. Teachers described the process as meaningful and joyful, reporting changes in their teaching practices, such as incorporating more student choice and wonder.

Table 21. Measure Dashboard for Playfulness.

Dimension	Rating	Description
Impact	●●○ **Moderate**	Has a noticeable effect for some contexts or groups. Contributes meaningfully but not comprehensively
Quality of Evidence	●○○ **Low**	Based mostly on anecdote, theory, or limited data
Context Dependency	●●● **High**	Highly dependent on specific cultural, institutional, or socioeconomic contexts; effectiveness is limited outside of these
Sustainability	●●○ **Moderate**	Some integration into structures or culture, but still somewhat dependent on leadership or budget
Teacher Voice	●●● **High**	Teachers co-design, adapt, and lead the initiative; their professional knowledge is central
Implementation Feasibility	●●○ **Moderate**	Requires some planning, adjustment, or collaboration. Feasible with committed leadership and moderate resource input

4.4. CREATE A SHARED SENSE OF MEANING

4.4.1. Shared Values and Goals

When teachers work in environments where common values and goals are emphasized, they tend to experience greater satisfaction of their psychological needs, especially a stronger sense of belonging, autonomy, and competence. This, in turn, leads to higher job satisfaction. In various contexts, alignment between individual and school values is linked to reduced emotional exhaustion and a lower desire to leave the profession. Professional relationships, collaboration, and clear, school-wide frameworks also play an important role in mitigating burnout while boosting teachers' confidence in their abilities and encouraging retention. This entails these major insights: Alignment of values and goals enhances job satisfaction and decreases intentions to leave. Shared goals contribute to teachers feeling more meaningful, connected, and overall well. These conclusions arise from a variety of research methods and consistently point to a positive relationship between shared educational goals and teacher well-being.

> Literature reviewed: H. B. Fox et al., 2020; Liang et al., 2020; Naghieh et al., 2015; Nwoko et al., 2023; Ortan et al., 2021; Ross et al., 2011; Skaalvik & Skaalvik, 2011, 2023; Soini et al., 2010; Toikka & Tarnanen, 2024; Turner et al., 2022; Zhou et al., 2024.

4.4.1.1. Measure

Promote shared educational goals and aligned values for your school.

4.4.1.1.1. 3 Key Components

- **Collaboratively define and communicate shared values and goals**

  Actively involve teaching staff in shaping and reinforcing a clear, shared vision and meaningful goals to foster teachers' sense of belonging, autonomy, and collective efficacy.

- **Establish regular processes to reflect on and refine shared values and goals**

  Create opportunities for teachers and leaders to review, discuss, and adjust shared values and goals to ensure they remain relevant and meaningful to all staff.

- **Encourage teachers to voice and bridge value and goal differences**

  Create safe, structured opportunities for teachers who feel misaligned with school values to openly share their perspectives. Through collaborative dialogue, these differences can be explored and bridged, fostering a stronger sense of inclusion and shared purpose.

For Measure Dashboard, see Table 22.

4.4.1.2. Good-Practice Example

4.4.1.2.1. England: Strengthening Behaviour and Well-Being Through Shared School Culture St. John's C. of E. Primary School in Bradford offers a strong example of how creating a consistent, values-led school culture can improve student behaviour and well-being (Ambition Institute, 2024). After participating in Ambition Institute's Leading Behaviour and Culture programme, the headteacher initiated a thorough review of the school's behaviour systems alongside support from the trust. The team redefined their school's vision to 'Children and their families always come first.' This has become embedded in every aspect of school life. This vision became the lens through which all decisions are made, from classroom routines to staff interactions with students and families. Crucially, the leadership team worked with staff to develop a shared behaviour curriculum. This included defining a clear, predictable set of routines and key phrases to use across the school. Instead of generic instructions like 'calm down' or 'be quiet', staff used specific prompts

Table 22. Measure Dashboard for Shared Values and Goals.

Dimension	Rating	Description
Impact	●●● **High**	Strong potential to transform teacher well-being. Addresses key drivers and has a broad, lasting impact
Quality of Evidence	●●● **High**	Strong, consistent evidence from rigorous research (e.g. meta-analyses, randomized controlled trials, longitudinal studies). Widely accepted in the field
Context Dependency	●○○ **Low**	Works effectively across most educational settings with minimal or no adaptation; broadly transferable
Sustainability	●●○ **Moderate**	Some integration into structures or culture, but still somewhat dependent on leadership or budget
Teacher Voice	●●● **High**	Teachers co-design, adapt, and lead the initiative; their professional knowledge is central
Implementation Feasibility	●●○ **Moderate**	Requires some planning, adjustment, or collaboration. Feasible with committed leadership and moderate resource input

such as 'impress me by sitting ready', helping students know exactly what is expected of them. Behaviour expectations were actively taught, modelled, and rehearsed with students, including those with additional needs. The staff also embraced consistent routines, such as specific entry and exit procedures, transitions, and language cues, thereby creating a calm and structured learning environment. This cultural shift reduced behaviour incidents, strengthened relationships with students, and gave staff more time to focus on meaningful teaching. Notably, teachers reported increased confidence in managing behaviour, and the school saw improved well-being among students and staff.

4.4.2. Collective Job Crafting

Job crafting – that is, the proactive shaping of tasks and roles to better fit individual strengths and needs – can be a powerful way to enhance well-being by increasing psychological empowerment, boosting work engagement, and reducing burnout. In various work settings, brief job-crafting interventions have been shown to lower negative emotions while raising self-efficacy and perceptions of career development opportunities. Observational studies further link job crafting with greater career satisfaction and stronger psychological resources, helping employees to adapt and thrive in their roles.

Among teachers, both individual and collective job crafting consistently improve work engagement, job satisfaction, and teaching performance. Structured sessions designed for educators lead to heightened psychological empowerment and affective well-being. Teachers also report using job crafting as a vital strategy to maintain their well-being during difficult periods, such as times of crisis, enabling them to sustain motivation and resilience in their professional lives.

Importantly, collective job crafting offers a way for teams to reflect on and reframe their shared work. By coming together to adjust tasks, align responsibilities with strengths, and explore how their roles connect to a broader purpose, teachers can rediscover meaning in their work. This shared effort strengthens collegial bonds and fosters a deeper sense of purpose and collective identity.

> Literature reviewed: Alonso et al., 2019; Aulén et al., 2024; Bakker et al., 2015; Dreer, 2022; Hakanen et al., 2017; M. Kim & Beehr, 2017; Mushtaq & Mehmood, 2023; Tims et al., 2013; van den Heuvel et al., 2015; van Wingerden et al., 2016; Vogt et al., 2015.

4.4.2.1. Measure

Enable meaningful work through collective and individual job crafting.

4.4.2.1.1. 3 Key Components

- **Introduce job crafting as a concept for professional growth**

  Start by familiarizing staff with the idea of job crafting, specifically how teachers can reshape their tasks, relationships, and work mindset to align better with their strengths and values.

- **Facilitate collective job-crafting workshops**

  Organize guided team sessions where staff reflect together on how to adjust roles, collaborate differently, or introduce new practices that boost engagement.

- **Create structural conditions that enable job crafting**

  Ensure that timetables, workload distribution, and team structures are flexible enough to give teachers real opportunities to shape, design, and share their work.

For Measure Dashboard, see Table 23.

Table 23. Measure Dashboard for Collective Job Crafting.

Dimension	Rating	Description
Impact	●●● **High**	Strong potential to transform teacher well-being. Addresses key drivers and has a broad, lasting impact
Quality of Evidence	●●● **High**	Strong, consistent evidence from rigorous research (e.g. meta-analyses, randomized controlled trials, longitudinal studies). Widely accepted in the field
Context Dependency	●●○ **Moderate**	Requires some adaptation but can function in several settings; effectiveness depends on moderately specific conditions (e.g. type of school)
Sustainability	●●● **High**	Embedded in institutional routines or culture; self-sustaining with minimal additional support
Teacher Voice	●●● **High**	Teachers co-design, adapt, and lead the initiative; their professional knowledge is central
Implementation Feasibility	●●○ **Moderate**	Requires some planning, adjustment, or collaboration. Feasible with committed leadership and moderate resource input

4.4.2.2. Good-Practice Example

4.4.2.2.1. England: Teachers Recraft Workload Collectively At Prince Henry's Grammar School in Otley, teachers and leaders came together for a whole-school 'workload review' built around a simple but powerful question: 'Do I really need to do this?' (C. Smith, 2018). Through collective reflection, staff identified unnecessary tasks and agreed on new routines to reduce pressure while maintaining high standards. They scrapped nonessential reports, dropped the requirement for detailed lesson plans in every observation, and sharply limited marking demands. For instance, written assessment was reduced to just one detailed marking task per subject each half-term, with class time set aside for students to act on feedback. Teachers reported that these changes freed them from excessive busywork, allowing for more focus on meaningful instruction. One teacher described the reforms as 'instrumental in maintaining the high standards that we want to provide for our students' (C. Smith, 2018, para. 17). By collaborating across the school, staff collectively crafted their environment.

4.5. NURTURE AND CELEBRATE TEACHER AND SCHOOL ACHIEVEMENTS

4.5.1. Collective Efficacy

Across diverse school systems, collective efficacy – that is, teachers' shared belief in their group's capacity to positively influence students – emerges as a powerful force for well-being. It fuels satisfaction, buffers against burnout, and cultivates a work environment where teachers feel energized, supported, and purposeful.

Research from seven countries, spanning a variety of educational levels and cultural contexts, consistently links collective efficacy to higher job satisfaction and improved psychological well-being among teachers. In schools where collective efficacy is strong, staff report greater optimism about their work, stronger emotional resilience, and a sense of belonging that helps sustain motivation even in difficult conditions. These schools often display an atmosphere of collegial trust, open communication, and a shared commitment to meaningful goals.

Collective efficacy fosters collegiality and collaboration, enhances perceptions of fairness, strengthens professional identity, and increases the perceived meaning of work. These dynamics, in turn, lower emotional exhaustion and build positive engagement.

Particularly striking is the consistency of these findings. Whether in urban schools or rural settings, among early-career teachers or veteran staff, the presence of strong collective efficacy correlates with better mental health, reduced stress, and higher motivation. Unlike some other forms of support, collective efficacy shows no signs of backfiring or producing unintended negative effects. Instead, it acts as a stabilizing and uplifting influence.

Literature reviewed: Buonomo et al., 2020; Caprara et al., 2003; Guidetti et al., 2018; Herrera et al., 2022; Klassen, 2010; Lei, 2024; Skaalvik & Skaalvik, 2019; Strahan née Brown et al., 2018; Yurt, 2022.

4.5.1.1. Measure

Build and sustain collective efficacy.

4.5.1.1.1. 3 Key Components

- **Facilitate structured peer collaboration**

  Create purposeful opportunities for teachers to co-plan, co-teach, co-reflect, or co-evaluate their work. Use team teaching, lesson study, or inquiry groups to foster a sense of joint ownership of student success. Collective problem-solving reinforces the belief that 'we can do this together'.

- **Collect and share student impact stories**

  Invite and collect meaningful expressions of gratitude and success, such as student letters, reflective essays, and alumni stories, and share them regularly with staff. This practice highlights the school's collective effort in shaping students' lives and strengthens the shared sense of purpose among educators.

  Use systematic data to illustrate progress

  Regularly share evidence of student growth and school improvements linked to teacher team efforts. Concrete proof of impact fuels motivation and belief.

For Measure Dashboard, see Table 24.

4.5.1.2. Good-Practice Example

4.5.1.2.1. Hawaii: Impact Teams for Improving Learning in Three Core Subjects The Sanford B. Dole Middle School located in Honolulu intentionally built teacher collaboration teams (referred to as 'impact teams') to

Table 24. Measure Dashboard for Collective Efficacy.

Dimension	Rating	Description
Impact	●●● **High**	Strong potential to transform teacher well-being. Addresses key drivers and has a broad, lasting impact
Quality of Evidence	●●● **High**	Strong, consistent evidence from rigorous research (e.g. meta-analyses, randomized controlled trials, longitudinal studies). Widely accepted in the field
Context Dependency	●●○○ **Low**	Works effectively across most educational settings with minimal or no adaptation; broadly transferable
Sustainability	●●○ **Moderate**	Some integration into structures or culture, but still somewhat dependent on leadership or budget
Teacher Voice	●●● **High**	Teachers co-design, adapt, and lead the initiative; their professional knowledge is central
Implementation Feasibility	●●○ **Moderate**	Requires some planning, adjustment, or collaboration. Feasible with committed leadership and moderate resource input

co-plan instruction and monitor student learning (The Core Collaborative, 2025). Teachers across the English, mathematics, and science departments meet in regular professional learning communities using structured 'analysis of evidence' and 'check-in' protocols to review student work, calibrate grading, and set learning goals. Staff co-constructed clear learning targets and success criteria with students, and then gathered formative assessment data to track progress. By the end of the school year, the school reported significant student gains. For example, overall proficiency rose by +4% in mathematics, +8% in English, and +12% in science. As a consequence, teachers noted a 'culture of collective efficacy' as they saw their collaborative strategies yielding measurable results.

4.5.2. Achievement Motivation

Achievement motivation, when supported and autonomous, consistently contributes to higher employee well-being across global work environments. In sectors ranging from education and retail to banking and public service, employees who are motivated by a desire to improve, master their tasks, and reach meaningful goals tend to experience enhanced vitality, engagement, and professional fulfilment. In Indonesia, Norway, and Pakistan, large-scale studies have shown that employees with strong achievement motivation demonstrate higher work effort, more positive affect, and a greater sense of progress in their roles. These benefits are most pronounced when motivation is self-directed and reinforced by the work environment, such as through empowering leadership, clear development opportunities, and recognition of meaningful accomplishments.

In the educational sector, this dynamic takes on particular relevance. Empirical findings show that teachers driven by genuine interest or internalized values consistently report greater job satisfaction, heightened vitality, and lower emotional exhaustion. Conversely, when achievement striving is driven by external pressure or fear of failure, and especially when teachers feel unsupported, stress and burnout become more likely. High achievement motivation, in the absence of adequate resources or recognition, can erode well-being over time. Supportive environments play a critical moderating role. Leadership that fosters autonomy, encourages constructive goal setting, and creates an emotionally safe culture helps teachers sustain motivation without compromising their health.

One key enabler across these contexts is the regular celebration of success, both small and large. When leaders actively acknowledge teachers' efforts and highlight everyday wins, such as positive student feedback or overcoming a classroom challenge, it reinforces a sense of purpose and psychological safety. This practice not only affirms the value of their work but also helps convert internal drive into resilience. When achievement is visible, shared, and meaningfully supported, it becomes a sustaining force for motivation.

> Literature reviewed: Bardach & Klassen, 2021; Bass, 1995; Chowdhury, 2007; Collie, 2014; Cuevas et al., 2018; Dysvik & Kuvaas, 2012; Jepson & Forrest, 2006; Lestari et al., 2023; Mahenthiran Aloysius & Christy, 2012; Makki & Abid, 2017; Morgan et al., 2007; Nie et al., 2014; Ololube, 2006; Raza et al., 2015; Rundle-Gardiner & Carr, 2005; Tutar et al., 2011; Wagner et al., 2015; H. Wang et al., 2016.

4.5.2.1. Measure

Foster healthy achievement motivation.

4.5.2.1.1. 3 Key Components

- **Celebrate big and small successes**

  Intentionally recognize and highlight a wide range of teacher achievements, from instructional innovations to positive student feedback. Public acknowledgements in staff meetings, newsletters, or informal gatherings reinforce intrinsic motivation and help teachers feel that their efforts are seen and valued.

- **Normalize diverse definitions of success**

  Communicate that success includes not only test scores or external validation, but also growth in student relationships, collaboration, and personal mastery. This helps teachers internalize healthier and more sustainable achievement standards.

- **Acknowledge effort and progress, not just outcomes**

  Reinforce that effort, experimentation, and reflective practice are valid achievements, especially during challenging periods or innovation processes.

For Measure Dashboard, see Table 25.

4.5.2.2. Good-Practice Example

4.5.2.2.1. Singapore: Celebrating Success to Support Teacher Motivation At St. Anthony's Canossian Secondary School, widely referred to as a 'happy school', leaders take an active role in supporting teacher well-being by fostering a culture of appreciation (National Institute of Education, 2021). Teachers are regularly asked what kind of support they need, and every

Table 25. Measure Dashboard for Achievement Motivation.

Dimension	Rating	Description
Impact	●●● **High**	Strong potential to transform teacher well-being. Addresses key drivers and has a broad, lasting impact
Quality of Evidence	●●● **High**	Strong, consistent evidence from rigorous research (e.g. meta-analyses, randomized controlled trials, longitudinal studies). Widely accepted in the field
Context Dependency	●○○ **Low**	Works effectively across most educational settings with minimal or no adaptation; broadly transferable
Sustainability	●●○ **Moderate**	Some integration into structures or culture, but still somewhat dependent on leadership or budget
Teacher Voice	●●○ **Moderate**	Some consultation with teachers, but limited decision-making power
Implementation Feasibility	●●● **High**	Easy to implement; minimal resources or barriers. Can be adopted with little disruption to daily practice

success, no matter how small, is publicly acknowledged. Staff meetings include celebrations of even modest wins, such as receiving a thank-you note from a parent. These intentional practices encourage teachers to notice and affirm one another's contributions, reinforcing a strong sense of belonging and shared purpose. By valuing both professional achievements and interpersonal appreciation, the school cultivates an emotionally supportive environment that helps sustain motivation and well-being.

5

EMPOWERING TEACHERS TO THRIVE

When considering teacher well-being at the individual level, it is important to use a framework that captures the complexity of human experience rather than reducing it to isolated stressors or surface-level indicators. Teachers are professionals who respond to policies and workloads; yet, they are also individuals with personal values, emotions, aspirations, and social contexts. Ryff's (1989) model of psychological well-being offers a particularly useful conceptual view because it integrates both emotional and functional aspects of well-being, enabling an understanding of what helps teachers thrive. The model outlines six interrelated dimensions (see Fig. 5).

(1) Self-acceptance involves recognizing and valuing oneself, including past successes, mistakes, and growth as a teacher, enabling confidence and self-worth despite professional challenges.

(2) Positive relations with others refer to building strong, trusting connections with colleagues, students, and the wider school community, which support emotional resilience and open collaboration.

(3) Autonomy relates to the ability to navigate and balance professional independence within the constraints of external demands, enabling teachers to make meaningful choices aligned with their personal and pedagogical values while adapting their practice to students' needs.

(4) Environmental mastery is about managing the professional environment effectively by balancing workload, resources, and expectations to support both student learning and personal well-being.

(5) Purpose relates to having meaningful goals and a clear sense of direction in one's work, such as a deep commitment to student growth or social impact.

(6) Finally, personal growth is the ongoing pursuit of new skills, understanding, and self-improvement, in which challenges are embraced as opportunities for development both professionally and personally.

Together, these dimensions provide a rich, nuanced picture of well-being that acknowledges the lived experiences of teachers and helps guide strategies for sustaining them in their work. Moreover, the model can serve as a valuable reflective template for teachers to assess their own well-being across these six dimensions. By identifying strengths and areas for growth, teachers can develop personalized strategies to enhance their well-being. This approach encourages ongoing self-awareness and intentional efforts to improve specific

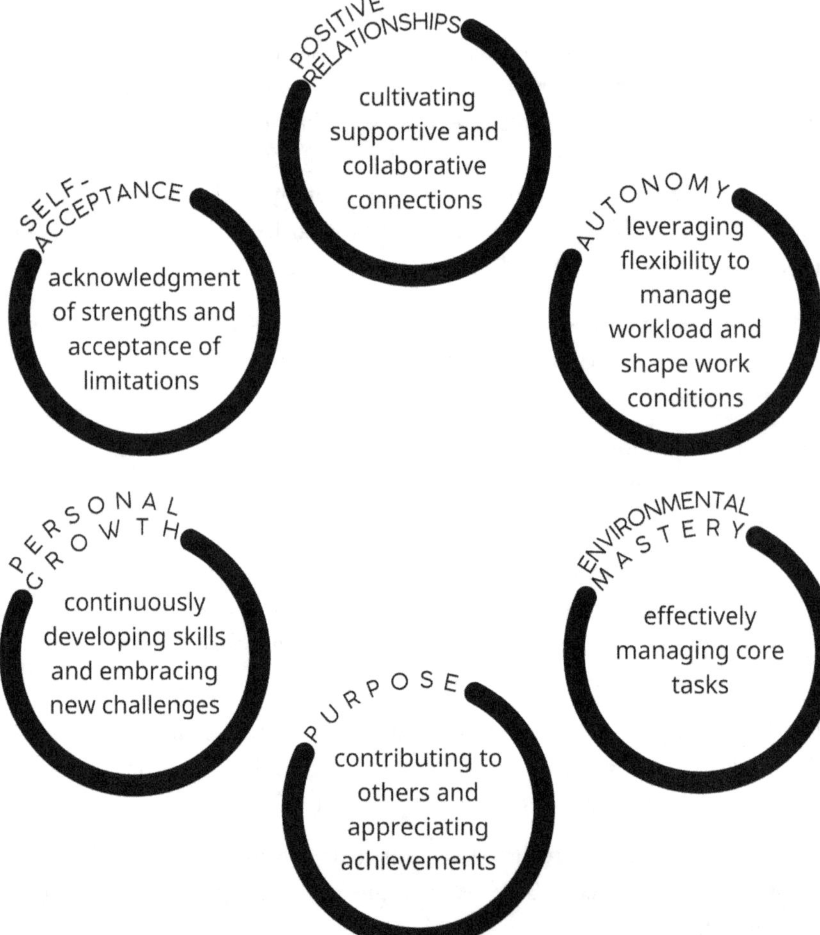

Fig. 5. Model of Psychological Well-Being by Ryff (1989). Figure Created by the Author.

aspects of their professional and personal lives, ultimately supporting a more sustainable and fulfilling teaching career.

The following subsections gather evidence about what teachers can change or prioritize with respect to their well-being. Using Ryff's (1989) model of psychological well-being, these are organized into measures that cultivate self-acceptance, foster positive relationships, help navigate autonomy, enhance environmental mastery, cultivate a clear sense of purpose, and encourage growth. The following suggestions are grounded in theory and current research findings. If certain aspects appear to be missing, it may be due to a lack of empirical investigation or inconclusive evidence regarding their effectiveness.

5.1. CULTIVATE SELF-ACCEPTANCE

5.1.1. Self-Compassion

Self-compassion is the practice of treating yourself with the same kindness, understanding, and patience that you would offer to a friend when facing mistakes, setbacks, or personal struggles. Practising self-compassion appears to lessen stress, anxiety, and burnout among teachers while enhancing emotional regulation and professional well-being. Quantitative studies (including randomized controlled trials) report significant negative correlations between self-compassion and indicators of stress. One 8-week Compassionate Mind Training for Teachers showed significant reductions in burnout and improvements in job satisfaction. Qualitative accounts from teachers corroborate these findings, noting that self-compassion fosters emotional recovery, self-awareness, and autonomy-supportive teaching practices. Institutional support and explicit training emerge as key factors in realizing these benefits, as evidenced by studies conducted across diverse cultural and educational settings.

Literature reviewed: Abbas et al., 2025; Awwad-Tabry, 2024; Awwad-Tabry & Levkovich, 2024; Gibbons & Newberry, 2022; Mairitsch et al., 2023; Matos et al., 2022; Moè & Katz, 2020; O'Hara-Gregan, 2023; Rajabi & Ghezelsefloo, 2020.

5.1.1.1. Measure

Practice self-compassion by treating yourself with the same kindness, patience, and understanding that you extend to others, especially when facing setbacks, mistakes, or stress.

5.1.1.1.1. 3 Key Components

- **Reframe with self-kindness**

  At the end of the day, replace harsh self-criticism with a compassionate reframe. Recognize challenges without judgement and acknowledge your effort, even when outcomes fall short.

- **Calibrate through shared humanity**

  Remind yourself that difficulties in teaching are part of the professional experience. Exchange struggles by connecting with colleagues' stories, professional communities, or reflective groups that highlight common challenges.

- **Support yourself with compassionate choices**

  Identify and follow through on one tangible action each day that reduces stress or restores energy, such as leaving school on time, taking a short walk, simplifying lesson preparation, or asking a colleague to share resources.

For Measure Dashboard, see Table 26.

Table 26. Measure Dashboard for Self-Compassion.

Dimension	Rating	Description
Impact	●●○ **Moderate**	Has a noticeable effect for some contexts or groups. Contributes meaningfully but not comprehensively
Quality of Evidence	●●● **High**	Strong, consistent evidence from rigorous research (e.g. meta-analyses, randomized controlled trials, longitudinal studies). Widely accepted in the field
Quality of Evidence	●●○ **Moderate**	Some research support, possibly from case studies or correlational data. Promising but not conclusive
Context Dependency	●●○ **Moderate**	Requires some adaptation but can function in several settings; effectiveness depends on moderately specific conditions (e.g. type of school)
Sustainability	●●○ **Moderate**	Some integration into structures or culture, but still somewhat dependent on leadership or budget
Teacher Voice	●●● **High**	Teachers co-design, adapt, and lead the initiative; their professional knowledge is central
Implementation Feasibility	●●○ **Moderate**	Requires some planning, adjustment, or collaboration. Feasible with committed leadership and moderate resource input

5.1.1.2. Good-Practice Example

5.1.1.2.1. India: Compassion Training for Teachers. In India, compassion-based training programmes have supported teachers in managing stress and reducing self-criticism. In Dharamshala, Tibetan school educators participated in SEE Learning and Cognitively-Based Compassion Training, where many admitted being overly harsh on themselves when lessons did not go as planned (Staff Editor, 2024). Through guided practice, they learned to show self-kindness without guilt, which improved their emotional resilience, classroom presence, and collegial support. A similar initiative in Patna engaged government school teachers and trainers from tribal, rural, and urban communities (P. Singh, 2024). Participants reflected on how excessively critical they had been of their own performance but found that cultivating compassion allowed them to manage their work without feeling overwhelmed, strengthen their teaching relationships, and foster more inclusive classrooms.

5.1.2. Optimism

Research from several countries shows that optimism supports teacher well-being, with evidence spanning Germany, Switzerland, Portugal, Romania, Türkiye, and Iran. Teachers who report higher levels of optimism tend to experience greater job satisfaction, stronger work engagement, and improved overall life satisfaction. Optimism is also linked to lower rates of burnout and fewer exhaustion symptoms, pointing to its protective role against workplace stress. Importantly, the benefits of optimism are not limited to emotional health; teachers with an optimistic outlook also report fewer physical health complaints, including musculoskeletal and voice-related problems.

The positive impact of optimism often operates through indirect pathways. Optimistic teachers are more likely to engage in proactive coping strategies, which help sustain work engagement. Optimism also supports self-efficacy, enabling teachers to feel more capable and effective in their roles.

> Literature reviewed: Borralho et al., 2025; Kun & Gadanecz, 2019; Magyar-Moe, 2014; Marcionetti & Castelli, 2022; Mavi et al., 2024; McLean et al., 2020; Mikus & Teoh, 2021; Soykan et al., 2019; Stănculescu, 2014; Zhou et al., 2024.

5.1.2.1. Measure

Develop habits that actively build and sustain optimism in your daily work.

5.1.2.1.1. 3 Key Components

- **Dispute unhelpful thoughts**

  Notice pessimistic beliefs and actively reframe them into balanced, constructive perspectives that support problem-solving and growth.

- **Transform setbacks**

  Acknowledge disappointments without judgement, then identify new possibilities or small steps forward that move you towards opportunity.

- **Set daily highlights**

  At the start of each day, choose one positive aspect to notice – whether it's a student's effort, a collegial interaction, or a personal achievement. When it occurs, fully savour the moment to strengthen your awareness of what is working well.

For Measure Dashboard, see Table 27.

5.1.2.2. Good-Practice Example

5.1.2.2.1. United States: Teacher-Led Positive Mindset Book Study. Individual teachers can use optimism practices to revive their passion. One notable

Table 27. Measure Dashboard for Optimism.

Dimension	Rating	Description
Impact	●●○ **Moderate**	Has a noticeable effect for some contexts or groups. Contributes meaningfully but not comprehensively
Quality of Evidence	●●○ **Moderate**	Some research support, possibly from case studies or correlational data. Promising but not conclusive
Context Dependency	●○○ **Low**	Works effectively across most educational settings with minimal or no adaptation; broadly transferable
Sustainability	●●● **High**	Embedded in institutional routines or culture; self-sustaining with minimal additional support
Teacher Voice	●●● **High**	Teachers co-design, adapt, and lead the initiative; their professional knowledge is central
Implementation Feasibility	●●● **High**	Easy to implement; minimal resources or barriers. Can be adopted with little disruption to daily practice

example is a Wisconsin elementary teacher who shared how a simple book study transformed her school's climate (Watson, 2017a). After nearly burning out, the teacher discovered Angela Watson's *Unshakeable: 20 Ways to Enjoy Teaching Every Day ... No Matter What.* She organized a staff book study around *Unshakeable* (for professional development credit) and subsequently reported that 'our school has started so positive this year' (Watson, 2017a, para. 4). The teacher attributed the turnaround entirely to the collective study of the optimistic principles from the book. This grassroots example underscores how optimism can be integrated into a school's routine to boost well-being.

5.2. NURTURE POSITIVE RELATIONSHIPS

5.2.1. Emotional Intelligence

Thriving as a teacher depends on understanding your own emotions and being aware of the feelings of those around you. This is where emotional intelligence, the ability to recognize, understand, and manage your own emotions while responding effectively to the emotions of others, becomes essential. Emotional intelligence relates consistently to teacher well-being across several domains. For example, one study found a strong positive correlation between overall emotional intelligence and psychological well-being, while another reported associations between emotional intelligence and work engagement, job satisfaction, and a negative correlation with burnout. A further study noted that teachers who naturally tend to recognize and manage their emotions (higher trait emotional intelligence) experience lower levels of burnout. In the affective and physical domains, higher emotional intelligence was linked to reduced stress, anxiety, and psychosomatic complaints, and specific dimensions such as clarity and repair were shown to bolster positive affect. Mediating and moderating factors, such as perseverance, social support, teaching experience, and happiness, appear to shape these associations, with one report indicating that the interplay between emotional intelligence and happiness explained 41% of the differences in job satisfaction.

At the same time, the teaching profession often requires managing emotions in ways that are not fully genuine. For example, teaching often requires showing calm, encouragement, or enthusiasm even when teachers do not feel it. This is captured by the concept of emotional labour, which refers to the process of managing feelings and expressions to fulfil the emotional requirements of a job. Research on teachers' emotional labour shows a nuanced impact on well-being depending on the strategy employed. Surface acting, the masking or faking of emotions, tends to increase burnout and emotional exhaustion, whereas deep acting, the modifying of internal feelings to align with required emotions, is associated with improved well-being and lower exhaustion. Expressing naturally felt emotions generally does not significantly affect well-being, while emotional dissonance, the conflict between felt and expressed emotions, is linked to negative outcomes.

Contextual factors can shape these effects. Social support, teaching self-efficacy, optimism, emotional intelligence, and clear organizational policies can buffer the negative effects of surface acting and enhance the benefits of deep acting.

For the individual teacher, this means that cultivating emotional intelligence, fostering supportive relationships, and developing strategies to manage emotions thoughtfully are key ways to maintain well-being and thrive professionally.

Literature reviewed: Akram et al., 2020; Avsec et al., 2009; Carey & Sutton, 2024; Cece et al., 2021; D'Amico et al., 2020; Dias & Arachchige, 2014; Dreer-Goethe, 2025d; Fernández-Berrocal et al., 2017; Fiorilli et al., 2019; Jennings & Greenberg, 2009; Kamboj & Garg, 2021; Karakus, Toprak, et al., 2024; Kinman et al., 2011; Murturi, 2024; Näring et al., 2006; Peláez-Fernández et al., 2021; Peng et al., 2023; Philipp & Schüpbach, 2010; Rasheed-Karim, 2020; Tuxford & Bradley, 2014; H. Wang et al., 2021.

5.2.1.1. Measure

Strengthen emotional intelligence through reflective, mindful, and social–emotional practices.

5.2.1.1.1. 3 Key Components

- **Acknowledge and respect emotional boundaries**

  Notice and acknowledge your emotions in the moment without judgement, labelling what you feel and allowing it to exist. At the same time, define clear boundaries for emotionally heavy issues. Decide which situations you will address personally and which you will escalate or hand off.

- **Practice empathy through perspective-taking exercises**

  Regularly engage in activities that encourage understanding others' emotions and viewpoints. This could include role-playing scenarios or discussing case studies that highlight diverse emotional responses.

- **Define display rules and prepare emotion scripts**

  Identify the emotions you want to be known for (e.g. curiosity, warmth) and create short scripts for common challenging situations, such as off-task behaviour or mistakes (e.g. 'I can see you're frustrated. Let's take two minutes and try again!'). Using scripts regularly helps automate positive emotional responses and reinforces beneficial self-regulation.

For Measure Dashboard, see Table 28.

5.2.1.2. Good-Practice Example

5.2.1.2.1. United States: Encouraging Teachers to Disclose Something Others Might Not Know. In Baltimore, the Happy Teacher Revolution has cultivated a supportive community where educators can openly share their personal challenges (Stark et al., 2022). During a peer support meeting, a music teacher encouraged participants to disclose something that others might not know about them. This prompt led to an immediate and heartfelt outpouring,

Table 28. Measure Dashboard for Emotional Intelligence.

Dimension	Rating	Description
Impact	●●● **High**	Strong potential to transform teacher well-being. Addresses key drivers and has a broad, lasting impact
Quality of Evidence	●●● **High**	Strong, consistent evidence from rigorous research (e.g. meta-analyses, randomized controlled trials, longitudinal studies). Widely accepted in the field
Context Dependency	●●○ **Moderate**	Requires some adaptation but can function in several settings; effectiveness depends on moderately specific conditions (e.g. type of school)
Sustainability	●●○ **Moderate**	Some integration into structures or culture, but still somewhat dependent on leadership or budget
Teacher Voice	●●● **High**	Teachers co-design, adapt, and lead the initiative; their professional knowledge is central
Implementation Feasibility	●●○ **Moderate**	Requires some planning, adjustment, or collaboration. Feasible with committed leadership and moderate resource input

with many teachers revealing struggles. One participant shared, 'I have really bad anxiety' (para. 20), a sentiment echoed by several others. This candid exchange fostered a sense of solidarity and empathy among the group, highlighting the importance of creating spaces where educators can be vulnerable and receive mutual support.

5.2.2. Elevation

Elevation is a special positive emotion that people experience when they witness excellence or acts of generosity, compassion, or courage in others. These observations often motivate action. People who feel elevated often want to imitate the good behaviour they have witnessed, improve their own skills, and help or support others. Research shows that elevation can lead to increased altruism, such as volunteering, helping strangers, or showing everyday kindness.

In the workplace, elevation can enhance well-being and teamwork. Witnessing acts of kindness, ethical leadership, or collaboration can inspire employees to support colleagues, act with integrity, and strengthen social connections. This not only fosters cooperation and a positive work environment but also boosts job satisfaction and resilience to stress.

For teachers, elevation can play a powerful role in their professional well-being. One study found that when preservice teachers observe experienced educators demonstrating compassion, ethical practice, and dedication in the classroom, it can positively influence their own sense of well-being. When experienced teachers report high levels of well-being, student teachers are more likely to feel inspired, motivated, and capable of adopting similar positive practices.

Context matters, however. Elevation is strongest when moral acts benefit others rather than the person performing them, highlighting its role in fostering selflessness. Compared to related emotions, gratitude tends to strengthen bonds with those who help us, while admiration motivates personal achievement, and elevation uniquely encourages moral growth, social openness, and prosocial action.

Literature reviewed: Algoe & Haidt, 2009; Chernikova, 2018; Clark & Newberry, 2019; Crissman, 2006; Dreer, 2023b; Pohling & Diessner, 2016; Schnall et al., 2010; Thomson & Siegel, 2017; Van Tongeren et al., 2018; Vianello et al., 2010; Waters, 2012; Williams, 2018.

5.2.2.1. Measure

Actively seek out and engage with exemplary teaching and moral actions in others.

5.2.2.1.1. 3 Key Components

- **Learn from exemplary colleagues**

  Focus on colleagues whose overall practice inspires professional and moral growth. Study their classroom strategies, decision-making, and teaching style to adopt best practices and improve your own teaching. This observation can occur in person or even through social media, where inspiring teaching practices and acts of kindness are shared.

- **Cultivate peer inspiration**

  Select three colleagues who each demonstrate a specific trait you admire (e.g. patience, empathy, dedication). Engage with them regularly through collaboration, discussion, or shared projects.

- **Act on inspiration**

  Transform the feeling of elevation into action by practising small prosocial behaviours, such as offering support to colleagues, mentoring students, or collaborating ethically on classroom initiatives.

For Measure Dashboard, see Table 29.

Table 29. Measure Dashboard for Elevation.

Dimension	Rating	Description
Impact	●●○ **Moderate**	Has a noticeable effect for some contexts or groups. Contributes meaningfully but not comprehensively
Quality of Evidence	●●○ **Moderate**	Some research support, possibly from case studies or correlational data. Promising but not conclusive
Context Dependency	●○○ **Low**	Works effectively across most educational settings with minimal or no adaptation; broadly transferable
Sustainability	●●● **High**	Embedded in institutional routines or culture; self-sustaining with minimal additional support
Teacher Voice	●●● **High**	Teachers co-design, adapt, and lead the initiative; their professional knowledge is central
Implementation Feasibility	●●● **High**	Easy to implement; minimal resources or barriers. Can be adopted with little disruption to daily practice

5.2.2.2. Good-Practice Example

5.2.2.2.1. United States: Driveway Messages of Kindness. During the COVID-19 pandemic-related school closures, two fifth-grade teachers in Minnesota turned to Facebook for inspiration. When they saw that colleagues in another state were writing chalk messages of encouragement on students' driveways, they felt uplifted and inspired (Wiita, 2021). This experience of elevation motivated them to share the idea with their own community. They spent hours visiting students' homes, writing positive notes such as 'You are loved' and 'We believe in you!' on sidewalks and driveways. Parents and children described feeling deeply cared for, and staff noted the ripple effect of kindness across the school. This example shows how witnessing compassion sparks elevation, which in turn motivates others to take prosocial action. Moreover, it highlights that elevation can occur not only through direct classroom observation but also by seeing acts of excellence and kindness shared via social media.

5.2.3. High-Quality Connections

High-quality connections are brief, meaningful moments between colleagues. Despite being spontaneous and informal conversations, both individuals feel seen, respected, and genuinely valued. These are the small yet powerful interactions, like a sincere 'How are you?' in the hallway or a brief caring conversation during a stressful day, which leaves both people feeling uplifted. Though fleeting, high-quality connections create ripples across school communities, fostering a culture of psychological safety, trust, and mutual regard. Research from Germany, France, Sweden, Japan, and Australia shows that in schools where these connections are frequent, teachers experience lower burnout, less emotional exhaustion, and greater job satisfaction. Simple rituals like shared check-ins, collaborative planning, or public appreciation boards help sustain these micro-moments of care. High-quality connections in the workplace can be fostered through three core strategies: respectful engagement, task enabling, and trusting. Respectful engagement means interacting with others in ways that show genuine care, presence, and appreciation, such as active listening, kind words, or simply acknowledging someone's effort. Task enabling involves helping others succeed by offering support, sharing resources, or removing obstacles, which strengthens collaboration and goodwill. Trusting includes taking the first step to show confidence in others, whether by being open, delegating responsibility, or seeking honest input.

Literature reviewed: Chhajer & Dutta, 2021; Dreer-Goethe, 2025c; Dutton, 2017; Dutton & Heaphy, 2003, 2005; Dutton & Ragins, 2007; Jacobsson et al., 2016; Prout et al., 2019; Rosales, 2016; Schön Persson et al., 2018; Sohail et al., 2023; Stephens et al., 2012; Temam et al., 2019; Tsuyuguchi, 2023; Turner et al., 2022.

5.2.3.1. Measure

Foster high-quality connections in your school by intentionally creating small moments of care, trust, and support with colleagues throughout your day.

5.2.3.1.1. 3 Key Components

- **Practise respectful engagement**

  Be fully present in conversations, even brief ones. Show genuine interest in how colleagues are doing, listen attentively, and acknowledge their efforts with kind words or gestures.

- **Enable others in their work**

  Look for small ways to make colleagues' tasks easier – whether by sharing resources, offering help, or simply removing an obstacle. Supporting others creates goodwill and strengthens collaboration.

- **Build trust through openness**

  Take small steps to show confidence in others. Invite honest input, share your own challenges, or delegate responsibility. When you extend trust, it encourages others to do the same.

For Measure Dashboard, see Table 30.

5.2.3.2. Good-Practice Example

5.2.3.2.1. Germany: The Power of Genuine Interest. During a school practicum, a student teacher reported a situation that altered well-being (Dreer-Goethe, 2025e). They experienced a challenging lesson in which the students were restless, loud, disrespectful, and chaotic. Afterwards, the student teacher was sitting alone in the teachers' lounge, feeling discouraged, when a colleague entered and asked with genuine interest how things were going. Grateful for the opportunity to share, the student teacher described the situation. The colleague responded by normalizing the experience, reassuring them that

Table 30. Measure Dashboard for High-Quality Connections.

Dimension	Rating	Description
Impact	●●○ **Moderate**	Has a noticeable effect for some contexts or groups. Contributes meaningfully but not comprehensively
Quality of Evidence	●●○ **Moderate**	Some research support, possibly from case studies or correlational data. Promising but not conclusive
Context Dependency	●○○ **Low**	Works effectively across most educational settings with minimal or no adaptation; broadly transferable
Sustainability	●●● **High**	Embedded in institutional routines or culture; self-sustaining with minimal additional support
Teacher Voice	●●● **High**	Teachers co-design, adapt, and lead the initiative; their professional knowledge is central
Implementation Feasibility	●●● **High**	Easy to implement; minimal resources or barriers. Can be adopted with little disruption to daily practice

they were not the only one who had difficulties with this class, and offering practical advice for handling such moments. The student teacher emphasized that, despite not knowing the colleague beforehand, even this brief interaction had a profoundly positive impact on their well-being. They felt taken seriously, understood, and supported, which reduced feelings of isolation and created a sense of psychological safety. The caring gesture strengthened collegial bonds and left them feeling relieved and grateful to have encountered such support during their practicum.

5.3. NAVIGATING AUTONOMY

5.3.1. Boundary Setting

Navigating autonomy in the workplace means setting boundaries. Being able to define when and how work happens allows individuals to manage their time and energy, supporting a sense of control and self-determination. Research with employees consistently shows that temporal segmentation, that is, establishing clear nonwork times or work–home boundaries, enhances well-being. Employees who maintain distinct boundaries report greater psychological detachment from work, improved relaxation, higher mastery experiences, and reduced emotional exhaustion. Field interventions and cross-sectional surveys suggest that clear time-based boundaries between work and nonwork periods improve post-work recovery. In addition, deliberately using mindfulness to mark the transition between work and nonwork, combined with supervisors who model healthy work–life practices, further reduces exhaustion and enhances life satisfaction. Conversely, blurred or technology-enabled boundaries, such as constant connectivity or inconsistent work demands, are associated with greater work–nonwork conflict, negative affect, and lower levels of happiness. Alignment between individual boundary preferences and actual practices also moderates these outcomes, highlighting the importance of personal agency in managing autonomy.

For teachers, maintaining clear professional–personal boundaries is not always easy, as much of their work extends beyond the classroom into home-based lesson preparation, constant communication with students and parents, and the personal affection invested in students. Teachers often have no official stopping point and could spend endless hours refining lesson plans or grading, which makes detachment challenging. Because of these demands and expectations, setting boundaries is essential for well-being. Teacher interviews and research reviews indicate that teachers who establish firm boundaries report lower levels of burnout and better mental health. Those who detach from work during nonwork hours experience less rumination, improved sleep quality, and reduced stress and depression symptoms. Mindful strategies, such as intentional transitions between work and home, and supportive school environments reinforce these benefits. Aligning boundaries with personal preferences promotes job satisfaction, reduces stress, and decreases turnover, while cultural and institutional contexts shape outcomes.

Literature reviewed: Becker et al., 2018; Binnewies et al., 2020; Büchler et al., 2020; Hahn & Dormann, 2013; Jusoh & Zhenni, 2025; Koch & Binnewies, 2015; Lutz et al., 2020; Persson & Thunman, 2017; Pluut & Wonders, 2020; Reinke & Gerlach, 2021; Rexroth et al., 2017; Tan & Urdan, 2025; Türktorun et al., 2020; Wepfer et al., 2017.

5.3.1.1. Measure

Set clear work–nonwork boundaries.

5.3.1.1.1. 3 Key Components

- **Define nonwork time**

  Decide on specific hours when work stops: no emails, phone calls, or preparations after that. If a task feels desperately unfinished, allow yourself a small, fixed extra window (e.g. 30 minutes) to complete it, but use this option no more than twice per week to protect your personal time.

- **Use mindful transitions**

  Build small rituals between work and personal time, such as a short walk, a transition playlist, or a technology pause. Choose small acts that signal the end of work and help create a clear mental separation.

- **Align practices with preferences**

  Regularly reflect on your ideal balance and adjust your daily routines as life circumstances change, such as family demands or special projects.

For Measure Dashboard, see Table 31.

5.3.1.2. Good-Practice Examples

5.3.1.2.1. United States: A Teacher's Boundary Strategy. A remote teacher in the United States shared how she negotiated clear boundaries with both her school and her students (Hickman, 2025). She communicated fixed work hours, specifying when she would be available for questions or feedback, and made it clear that lessons and emails outside these times were optional. By doing so, she created structured expectations that allowed her to focus on teaching during set hours while protecting her personal time. This practice

Table 31. Measure Dashboard for Boundary Setting.

Dimension	Rating	Description
Impact	●●● **High**	Strong potential to transform teacher well-being. Addresses key drivers and has a broad, lasting impact
Quality of Evidence	●●○ **Moderate**	Some research support, possibly from case studies or correlational data. Promising but not conclusive
Context Dependency	●●○ **Moderate**	Requires some adaptation but can function in several settings; effectiveness depends on moderately specific conditions (e.g. type of school)
Sustainability	●●● **High**	Embedded in institutional routines or culture; self-sustaining with minimal additional support
Teacher Voice	●●● **High**	Teachers co-design, adapt, and lead the initiative; their professional knowledge is central
Implementation Feasibility	●●○ **Moderate**	Requires some planning, adjustment, or collaboration. Feasible with committed leadership and moderate resource input

helped reduce stress and maintain a sustainable balance between professional responsibilities and home life.

5.3.1.2.2. Singapore: Managing After-Hours Expectations. A secondary school teacher in Singapore shared her experience of parents contacting her outside of school hours, often expecting immediate responses (Min, 2024). She emphasized that unless it is a real emergency, such as a child being missing or injured, there is no issue that cannot wait until the next day. To manage these expectations, she and her colleagues set clear boundaries. They informed parents that teachers work until about 5.00 or 6.00 p.m. and requested that they respect these hours. Furthermore, they refrained from sharing personal phone numbers with parents and used official communication channels instead. By establishing and maintaining these boundaries, the teacher was able to protect her personal time and reduce stress.

5.3.2. Rest Breaks

Rest breaks are recognized as vital components of healthy work environments, offering benefits that extend beyond momentary relief. Across a variety of professions, short pauses during the workday have been shown to ease physical fatigue, reduce discomfort, and prevent the buildup of musculoskeletal strain. They also serve an important psychological function by lowering stress levels, restoring concentration, and enhancing energy. The timing, length, and nature of these breaks matter. Brief, restorative moments, whether stretching, walking, or simply stepping away from the task, support recovery without compromising productivity. Evidence from healthcare, office, and manual labour settings consistently highlights that both scheduled and employee-chosen breaks help restore resources, alleviate symptoms, and improve overall mood, with positive knock-on effects for job performance and interpersonal relations at work.

Within the teaching profession, these dynamics are particularly relevant. Research shows that incorporating a lunch break along with smaller pauses between lessons contributes meaningfully to reducing exhaustion and feelings of inadequacy among teachers. The impact is especially marked for older subject teachers, though class teachers often face structural barriers that limit opportunities for rest. In practice, many of the short breaks available are quickly absorbed by organizational duties, such as preparing the next lesson, moving between classrooms or buildings, and responding to student concerns, leaving little space for true recovery. Still, even informal or unplanned breaks have been found to play a critical role in sustaining resilience. These moments allow teachers to mentally detach, physically relax, and better manage the constant demands and uncertainties inherent in the profession. Taken together, the findings point to the fact that regular, meaningful breaks are essential for protecting teacher well-being and ensuring their capacity to meet the complex demands of the classroom.

> Literature reviewed: Albulescu et al., 2022; Blasche et al., 2016; Dababneh et al., 2001; Henning et al., 1997; Hunter & Wu, 2016; Kinnunen et al., 2019; Lindqvist & Nordänger, 2006; Lyubykh et al., 2022; O'Neill et al., 2022; Sianoja et al., 2018; Wendsche et al., 2016, 2017, 2023.

5.3.2.1. Measure

Prioritize restorative breaks during the school day.

5.3.2.1.1. 3 Key Components

- **Protect true recovery time**

  Differentiate between breaks used for organizational duties (lesson preparation, moving classrooms, addressing student needs) and those reserved for genuine rest, ensuring at least one pause each day supports relaxation or detachment.

- **Integrate small restorative practices**

  Integrate small restorative practices throughout the day, even during teaching. Plan lessons to include short breaks that ease strain, restore focus, and give you a moment out of the spotlight.

- **Adapt to context and needs**

  Reflect on your personal energy rhythms and teaching schedule to identify when breaks are most impactful, and adjust routines to maximize recovery within available opportunities.

For Measure Dashboard, see Table 32.

Table 32. Measure Dashboard for Rest Breaks.

Dimension	Rating	Description
Impact	●●● **High**	Strong potential to transform teacher well-being. Addresses key drivers and has a broad, lasting impact
Quality of Evidence	●●● **High**	Strong, consistent evidence from rigorous research (e.g. meta-analyses, randomized controlled trials, longitudinal studies). Widely accepted in the field
Context Dependency	●●○ **Moderate**	Requires some adaptation but can function in several settings; effectiveness depends on moderately specific conditions (e.g. type of school)
Sustainability	●●○ **Moderate**	Some integration into structures or culture, but still somewhat dependent on leadership or budget
Teacher Voice	●●○ **Moderate**	Some consultation with teachers, but limited decision-making power
Implementation Feasibility	●●○ **Moderate**	Requires some planning, adjustment, or collaboration. Feasible with committed leadership and moderate resource input

5.3.2.2. Good-Practice Examples

5.3.2.2.1. Finland: The Journey to Embracing Teacher Breaks. In Finnish schools, it is customary for every 45 minutes of instruction to be followed by a 15-minute recess. Students head outdoors to play, while teachers typically retreat to the staff lounge for coffee and conversation (Walker, 2014). When a US teacher first began teaching in Finland, he resisted the local custom of giving students and himself a 15-minute break after every 45 minutes of instruction. Following his US instincts, he tried doubling the teaching block to 1.5 hours and then offering a longer recess. The outcome was immediate – his students became restless and disengaged. Realizing the toll on both his students and himself, the teacher reverted to the Finnish rhythm of shorter, more frequent breaks. The difference was striking. Not only did the children return to class energized and focused, but the teacher found himself recharged too. Those lounge conversations over coffee with colleagues became a vital release valve, preventing burnout and restoring balance during the school day. Over time, he came to see these interludes not as lost instructional minutes but as essential investments in sustained attention, calm, and teacher well-being.

5.3.2.2.2. United States: Teachers Turn to Jigsaw Puzzles to Escape Toxic 'always-on' Culture.

An eighth-grade English teacher in Hartford, Connecticut, decided to reclaim her break time in a refreshingly simple and effective way: by bringing a partially completed jigsaw puzzle into the teachers' lounge (Klein, 2022). 'Everybody friggin' loves it', she said, noting that 'we finished 11 puzzles so far this year'. More than just idle distraction, the puzzle has helped shift lunchroom chatter away from incessant 'shop talk' and into a looser, more light-hearted headspace, giving teachers a much-needed mental breather during their hectic days.

5.3.3. Individual Job Crafting

Job crafting refers to the process by which teachers use their autonomy to actively adjust aspects of their work to better fit their strengths, interests, and preferences. This can involve shaping tasks (e.g. choosing to adjust the order of tasks), relationships (e.g. building stronger connections with colleagues who inspire and support), and perceptions of work (e.g. redefining what is considered part of the role and what not to take on). On an individual level, strategies may include seeking additional resources such as professional development opportunities, mentorship, or collaborative support from external partners. They may also involve embracing challenging demands by taking on new projects, experimenting with innovative teaching methods, or setting personal growth goals. Finally, strategies can focus on reducing hindering demands by reorganizing tasks, managing workload more efficiently, or setting boundaries to minimize stress. Job crafting has been consistently shown to support individual teacher well-being. Engaging in these strategies is associated with higher work engagement, enhanced psychological well-being, greater job satisfaction, and improved job performance. Research shows that by actively crafting their jobs, teachers can cultivate greater engagement, resilience, and relational quality, making it a practical approach to fostering individual well-being in diverse educational settings.

> Literature reviewed: Alonso et al., 2019; Aulén et al., 2024; Bakker et al., 2015; Dreer, 2022; Hakanen et al., 2017; M. Kim & Beehr, 2017; Mushtaq & Mehmood, 2023; Tims et al., 2013; van den Heuvel et al., 2015; van Wingerden et al., 2016; Vogt et al., 2015.

5.3.3.1. Measure

Take control of your work by actively shaping your tasks, relationships, and approach to teaching to better fit your strengths and interests.

5.3.3.1.1. 3 Key Components

- **Understand job crafting as a tool for your growth**

  Start by familiarizing yourself with the idea of job crafting. Reflect on how you can adjust your tasks, relationships, and mindset to align better with your strengths, interests, and values.

- **Reflect on your work and strengths**

  Think about which parts of your teaching energize you and which feel draining. Identify tasks, interactions, or routines you could adjust to make your work more meaningful and enjoyable.

- **Use your autonomy to shape your work environment**

  Leverage the flexibility you have in planning lessons, managing your classroom, and interacting with students and colleagues. Make intentional changes to your routines that better fit your preferences.

For Measure Dashboard, see Table 33.

Table 33. Measure Dashboard for Individual Job Crafting.

Dimension	Rating	Description
Impact	●●● **High**	Strong potential to transform teacher well-being. Addresses key drivers and has a broad, lasting impact
Quality of Evidence	●●● **High**	Strong, consistent evidence from rigorous research (e.g. meta-analyses, randomized controlled trials, longitudinal studies). Widely accepted in the field
Context Dependency	●●○ **Moderate**	Requires some adaptation but can function in several settings; effectiveness depends on moderately specific conditions (e.g. type of school)
Sustainability	●●● **High**	Embedded in institutional routines or culture; self-sustaining with minimal additional support
Teacher Voice	●●● **High**	Teachers co-design, adapt, and lead the initiative; their professional knowledge is central
Implementation Feasibility	●●○ **Moderate**	Requires some planning, adjustment, or collaboration. Feasible with committed leadership and moderate resource input

5.3.3.2. Good-Practice Example

5.3.3.2.1. Australia: How Teachers Reimagine Their Roles Through Job Crafting. An Australian study highlighted how teachers are finding creative ways to craft their jobs by weaving personal passions into lessons, building collaborative routines, and redefining their sense of purpose, creating richer, more engaging experiences for both themselves and their students (Slemp et al., 2023). One primary teacher, a card-game enthusiast, described how he incorporates his hobby into mathematics lessons:

> *I bring a lot of those card games into class with the kids and we find the maths in the games ... I think they can definitely sense my passion for the games and that makes them more excited. I've had quite a few parents say, 'My child now loves maths because of the way you play the games,' which is really nice. (para. 10)*

A secondary teacher explained how she often invited colleagues into her classroom:

> *I love saying to the other teachers, 'Hey, do you want to drop into my class because I think you'll like it' or 'This kid misses you, he hasn't seen you in ages, do you want to come swing by?' It's so nice to have other adults in the room ... And [for] teachers that you have really good relationships with, you can then model what a healthy relationship looks like to the kids. (para. 14)*

5.4. IMPROVE ENVIRONMENTAL MASTERY

5.4.1. Mastery Goals

The goals people set at work shape how they feel and how they perform. Goals give direction, influence motivation, and affect well-being in daily life. Among the different types of goals, mastery goals stand out because they focus on learning, improving, and developing competence rather than competing with others.

Employees who pursue mastery-approach goals (e.g. trying out new ways to explain difficult content) often develop stronger relationships with supervisors, perform better, and experience greater job satisfaction. They also tend to be more engaged in their work, particularly when they feel supported with the necessary resources. By contrast, mastery-avoidance goals (e.g. avoiding situations where they might not have an answer) are linked to detachment and fatigue, as they reduce opportunities for emotional support. These goals are less about striving to grow and more about trying not to fail, which can drain energy and motivation. Generally, the match between achievement goals, autonomy, and learning opportunities is especially important; when aligned, employees adjust more successfully to career transitions and report higher levels of well-being.

The same patterns are evident in teaching. Teachers with mastery-approach goals report greater job satisfaction, positive emotions, and overall life satisfaction, while work-avoidance goals undermine well-being. Their emotional responses to challenging student behaviour strongly influence their well-being, highlighting the importance of goal orientations in daily classroom life. The relationship between goals and well-being is reciprocal. That means mastery goals strengthen well-being, and well-being, in turn, reinforces mastery orientations, creating a cycle that sustains both professional effectiveness and personal fulfilment.

Literature reviewed: Ames & Archer, 1988; Benita & Matos, 2021; Butler, 2012; Forster et al., 2022; Gillet et al., 2012; Heidemeier & Wiese, 2014; Janssen & Van Yperen, 2004; Nagy et al., 2024; Page, 2005; Poortvliet et al., 2015; Rinas et al., 2020, 2023; Santos et al., 2012; Shim et al., 2013; van Dam et al., 2020; Watt & Richardson, 2020.

5.4.1.1. Measure

Set professional goals that focus on learning, growth, and continuous improvement rather than avoiding mistakes or comparing yourself to others.

5.4.1.1.1. 3 Key Components

- **Understand mastery goals as a path to growth**

  Recognize that mastery goals are about developing competence and improving over time. Reflect on how shifting your mindset from 'not failing' to 'getting better' can energize you and make your work more meaningful.

- **Choose goals that align with your values and interests**

  Focus on learning objectives and skill development that energize you and feel personally meaningful. Prioritize goals that you are intrinsically motivated to pursue and that enhance your sense of purpose and engagement in your work. Ensure that your goals reflect what matters most to you.

- **Incorporate challenge and skill stretch**

  Design goals that push your current abilities just enough to promote learning without causing burnout. Choose tasks that are slightly beyond your current comfort zone, such as experimenting with a new teaching strategy or engaging in a professional development activity.

For Measure Dashboard, see Table 34.

5.4.1.2. Good-Practice Example

5.4.1.2.1. England: Focusing on Mastery, Not Comparison. On a teacher blog, an educator reflected on the stress caused by constantly comparing her classroom to the 'Pinterest-perfect' images shared by others (Watson, 2017b). She described how this left her feeling as though her efforts were never enough, even when her teaching was effective. To protect her well-being, she chose to stop measuring herself against others and instead set mastery goals that suited her own practice. This meant focusing on what truly mattered for her students' learning and on making steady improvements in her own teaching, rather than striving for decorative displays or elaborate setups. By reframing her work in this way, she reported feeling less anxious, more purposeful, and more connected to the core of her role. Her story illustrates how avoiding social comparison and committing to self-referenced mastery goals can help teachers sustain both their motivation and their well-being.

Table 34. Measure Dashboard for Mastery Goals.

Dimension	Rating	Description
Impact	●●● **High**	Strong potential to transform teacher well-being. Addresses key drivers and has a broad, lasting impact
Quality of Evidence	●●● **High**	Strong, consistent evidence from rigorous research (e.g. meta-analyses, randomized controlled trials, longitudinal studies). Widely accepted in the field
Context Dependency	●●○ **Moderate**	Requires some adaptation but can function in several settings; effectiveness depends on moderately specific conditions (e.g. type of school)
Sustainability	●●● **High**	Embedded in institutional routines or culture; self-sustaining with minimal additional support
Teacher Voice	●●● **High**	Teachers co-design, adapt, and lead the initiative; their professional knowledge is central
Implementation Feasibility	●●● **High**	Easy to implement; minimal resources or barriers. Can be adopted with little disruption to daily practice

5.4.2. Conflict and Classroom Management

Schools are hubs of relationships and interactions every day, where conflicts naturally arise among colleagues, students, and teams. For teachers, learning to handle conflicts with colleagues, students, parents, and within teams is one of the most important skills for mastering the profession. How teachers manage these situations has a direct impact on their well-being and on their ability to carry out their work smoothly and effectively. Teachers who handle conflicts and classroom challenges effectively tend to feel less stressed, more confident, and more in control of their work. Using problem-solving approaches to address disagreements or challenges reduces stress and emotional exhaustion, while relying on dominating, compromising, or avoidance strategies can increase stress, burnout, and disengagement. Supportive colleagues and leaders who recognize emotions can help lessen these negative effects, and seeking help or building social support can protect against feelings of isolation and reduce turnover intentions.

In the classroom, the same patterns are clear. Teachers who rely on reactive strategies, responding only to problems as they arise, often feel more stressed and less able to manage their classrooms. By contrast, proactive strategies, including structured interventions and planning, increase teacher confidence, reduce stress, and improve overall well-being. Emotional resources matter too; teachers who maintain positive emotions and lower levels of exhaustion are better able to apply effective management practices. Consequently, well-being and management skills are closely intertwined; feeling well supports effective conflict and classroom management, while practising strong management skills reinforces confidence, reduces stress, and strengthens well-being.

> Literature reviewed: Clunies-Ross et al., 2008; Herman et al., 2017; Kennedy et al., 2021; Lauth-Lebens & Lauth, 2016; Leckey et al., 2016; Li et al., 2022; Marlow et al., 2015; Mennes et al., 2024; Seiza et al., 2015.

5.4.2.1. Measure

Develop effective conflict and classroom management practices while recognizing and respecting your personal limits.

5.4.2.1.1. 3 Key Components

- **Manage conflicts constructively**

  Use problem-solving approaches to address disagreements with colleagues, supervisors, or teams. Avoid dominating, compromising, or purely avoidance-based strategies, as they can increase stress and disengagement. Seek support when needed and cultivate a supportive work climate to buffer negative outcomes like burnout, absenteeism, and loneliness.

- **Strengthen classroom management proactively**

  Focus on proactive strategies that anticipate and prevent classroom challenges rather than simply reacting to issues as they arise. Structured routines, clear expectations, and consistent procedures enhance teacher self-efficacy, reduce stress, and improve classroom control.

- **Know your limits and prioritize well-being**

  Recognize when stress, exhaustion, or a high workload interfere with your ability to manage conflicts or maintain classroom control. Use breaks, delegate tasks when possible, and seek help to maintain balance. Understanding your limits helps prevent burnout and ensures that both classroom and conflict management practices remain effective over time.

For Measure Dashboard, see Table 35.

5.4.2.2. Good-Practice Examples

5.4.2.2.1. Ghana: Positive Discipline Through Play. In Ghana, a primary school teacher described how the stress of managing misbehaviour had

Table 35. Measure Dashboard for Conflict and Classroom Management.

Dimension	Rating	Description
Impact	●●● **High**	Strong potential to transform teacher well-being. Addresses key drivers and has a broad, lasting impact
Quality of Evidence	●●● **High**	Strong, consistent evidence from rigorous research (e.g. meta-analyses, randomized controlled trials, longitudinal studies). Widely accepted in the field
Context Dependency	●●○ **Moderate**	Requires some adaptation but can function in several settings; effectiveness depends on moderately specific conditions (e.g. type of school).
Sustainability	●●○ **Moderate**	Some integration into structures or culture, but still somewhat dependent on leadership or budget
Teacher Voice	●●○ **Moderate**	Some consultation with teachers, but limited decision-making power
Implementation Feasibility	●●○ **Moderate**	Requires some planning, adjustment, or collaboration. Feasible with committed leadership and moderate resource input

once led her to rely on corporal punishment, leaving her feeling discouraged and exhausted (Right to Play, 2025). After taking part in a programme that introduced play-based and learner-centred methods, she found that student behaviour improved and classroom discipline became less of a struggle. She reported feeling 'happier and more relaxed' (para. 12) as children became more engaged and respectful, which, in turn, restored her confidence and enjoyment in teaching. Her experience shows how adopting positive, participatory approaches can reduce stress, improve classroom climate, and strengthen teacher well-being.

5.4.2.2.2. United States: Proactive Routines Restore Balance. In an interview on the Shake Up Learning Show, a veteran educator reflects on the challenges of classroom stress and burnout (Bell, 2024). She explained that by shifting towards firm but positive classroom management strategies, including clear expectations, consistent routines, and positive reinforcement, she was able to create a calmer environment where students knew what to expect. This proactive approach helped her regain control of her classroom, reduce daily stress, and restore balance between work and personal life. She reported that the strategies saved time, reduced burnout, and allowed her to rediscover joy in teaching.

5.5. CLARIFY AND CONNECT WITH PURPOSE

5.5.1. Mentoring

Finding meaning and purpose in teaching often comes not only from working with students but also from contributing to the growth of colleagues. Mentoring represents a distinct professional role that allows teachers to step into positions of guidance, support, and leadership. Being a mentor can have a powerful positive impact on teacher well-being, offering opportunities for professional growth, enhanced confidence, and a stronger sense of belonging. When the mentoring relationship is characterized by trust, open communication, and mutual respect, mentors often report gains in work-related engagement, a greater sense of purpose, and a heightened feeling of achievement. They also experience emotional benefits, such as feeling valued, more connected to their professional community, and motivated by the chance to contribute to the development of others. In this way, mentoring not only supports the mentee but also reinforces the mentor's identity and satisfaction as an educator.

However, the effectiveness of mentoring also depends on external conditions. Factors such as dedicated time for regular interactions, access to targeted mentor training, and a supportive institutional culture significantly enhance the positive outcomes of mentoring. Conversely, when mentors face challenges such as strained or negative relationships with mentees, limited institutional support, or insufficient preparation for their roles, the experience can lead to frustration, heightened stress, and, in some cases, burnout.

> Literature reviewed: Abetang et al., 2020; Corrigan & Loughran, 2008; Dahal, 2023; Dreer-Goethe, 2023, 2025b; Hollweck, 2019; Kuhn et al., 2022; Oh et al., 2024; Orland-Barak, 2001; Richter et al., 2021; Thornton, 2025.

5.5.1.1. Measure

Perceive mentoring as a way to positively impact your own well-being while actively engaging in the development of the next generation of teachers.

5.5.1.1.1. 3 Key Components

- **Relive your achievements**

  Perceive mentoring as an opportunity to revisit the beginnings and successes of your teaching career. Reflecting on your own achievements while guiding a mentee reinforces your sense of professional competence, pride, and satisfaction.

- **Experience and appreciate growth in your mentee**

  Take time to notice and celebrate the progress your mentee makes, whether big or small. Seeing their development reinforces your sense of purpose and highlights the impact of your guidance.

- **Invest in the relationship**

  Build a professional partnership with your mentee by creating a foundation of trust, respect, and open communication. Set shared goals, provide constructive feedback, and celebrate progress together. A strong mentoring relationship fosters growth for both you and your mentee while also strengthening your connection to your professional community.

For Measure Dashboard, see Table 36.

Table 36. Measure Dashboard for Mentoring.

Dimension	Rating	Description
Impact	●●● **High**	Strong potential to transform teacher well-being. Addresses key drivers and has broad, lasting impact
Quality of Evidence	●●○ **Moderate**	Some research support, possibly from case studies or correlational data. Promising but not conclusive
Context Dependency	●○○ **Low**	Works effectively across most educational settings with minimal or no adaptation; broadly transferable
Sustainability	●●○ **Moderate**	Some integration into structures or culture, but still somewhat dependent on leadership or budget
Teacher Voice	●●● **High**	Teachers co-design, adapt, and lead the initiative; their professional knowledge is central
Implementation Feasibility	●●○ **Moderate**	Requires some planning, adjustment, or collaboration. Feasible with committed leadership and moderate resource input

5.5.1.2. Good-Practice Example

5.5.1.2.1. United States: Mentorship as a Pathway to Teacher Well-Being. An elementary art teacher at Truesdell Elementary School in Washington, D.C., exemplifies how mentorship has sustained his commitment to teaching (Grajeda, 2024). Starting his career as a Teach For America Corps member in Jacksonville, Florida, this teacher faced numerous challenges, including low pay, lack of experience, and overwhelming demands. Despite these obstacles, he remained in the profession for over a decade, primarily in underserved schools across multiple states. He attributes his perseverance to the strong relationships he built with fellow educators through mentorship, collegial support, and friendship. These connections provided not only practical guidance and feedback but also emotional support during difficult times. He reported,

> *Helping these new educators navigate their first year of teaching was one of the most rewarding experiences of my career. I saw myself in their struggles with classroom management and lesson planning, and I was eager to share the strategies that had helped me. Watching them grow as teachers and having a hand in their success reignited my passion for teaching. (para. 12)*

5.5.2. Gratitude

Teacher gratitude has emerged as a strong driver of well-being, consistently associated with higher life satisfaction, increased work engagement, and lower burnout across diverse countries. Educators who cultivate gratitude through reflecting on positive experiences – for example, by maintaining gratitude journals – tend to experience stronger subjective and psychological well-being. These effects are amplified when teachers perceive supportive job resources, strong social networks, and positive relationships with students, which help translate feelings of gratitude into meaningful professional and personal outcomes. While gratitude-based practices generally enhance well-being and buffer against burnout, their effects may be less pronounced in contexts of extreme adversity, highlighting that gratitude practices alone cannot mend the systemic stressors and structural issues individuals face.

Literature reviewed: Allen et al., 2024; Chan, 2010, 2011; Dreer, 2020; Howells, 2014; Jeliseh et al., 2025; Nicuţă et al., 2022; Rahm & Heise, 2019; Waters, 2012; Zheng et al., 2024.

5.5.2.1. Measure

Cultivate gratitude in your daily work practice.

5.5.2.1.1. 3 Key Components

- **Reflect on experiences that inspire gratitude**

  Regularly notice and record moments that evoke a sense of thankfulness, such as student progress, personal achievements, supportive interactions, or lessons learned from challenges.

- **Appreciate key professional relationships**

  Notice and be thankful for key professional relationships, like mentors, colleagues, and trusted contacts, reflecting on what makes these relationships meaningful. Express gratitude—for example, through handwritten or digital thank-you notes or small gestures of appreciation.

- **Engage in gratitude practices**

  Adopt research-backed gratitude practices such as 'counting blessings' journaling, the 'three good things' exercise and 'gratitude letters' or 'gratitude visits'.

For Measure Dashboard, see Table 37.

Table 37. Measure Dashboard for Gratitude.

Dimension	Rating	Description
Impact	●●● **High**	Strong potential to transform teacher well-being. Addresses key drivers and has a broad, lasting impact
Quality of Evidence	●●○ **Moderate**	Some research support, possibly from case studies or correlational data. Promising but not conclusive
Context Dependency	●●○ **Moderate**	Requires some adaptation but can function in several settings; effectiveness depends on moderately specific conditions (e.g. type of school)
Sustainability	●●● **High**	Embedded in institutional routines or culture; self-sustaining with minimal additional support
Teacher Voice	●●● **High**	Teachers co-design, adapt, and lead the initiative; their professional knowledge is central
Implementation Feasibility	●●● **High**	Easy to implement; minimal resources or barriers. Can be adopted with little disruption to daily practice

5.5.2.2. Good-Practice Example

5.5.2.2.1. South Africa: A Moment of Gratitude That Transformed Teaching. In South Africa, a young teacher at Maritzburg College in Pietermaritzburg (Natal) recalled the powerful influence of a mentor (Howells, 2024). Before entering the classroom, the mentor would pause, with eyes closed, almost in prayer, to consciously feel gratitude. He reminded himself that he was about to teach students who were 'brighter and more articulate' than he and who would one day achieve more. That humble ritual helped the mentor approach teaching as a privilege rather than a job. Over time, the mentee realized that while he could never match his mentor's effectiveness, learning to teach with thankfulness made his own teaching far more enjoyable. This intentional pause, grounded in humility and authentic appreciation, rendered gratitude not merely as a formality but as a deeply transformative daily practice.

5.6. ENGAGE IN PERSONAL GROWTH

5.6.1. Growth Mindset

A growth mindset, the belief that abilities can develop through effort, is associated with improved teacher well-being, including greater emotional resilience, life satisfaction, and reduced burnout and stress. However, this positive effect is influenced by specific moderating factors. Teachers with less experience benefit more from growth mindset beliefs, likely because early-career educators face steeper learning curves and higher stress levels. Cultural background also matters; the benefits of a growth mindset are stronger in collectivist cultures, where effort and persistence are more socially emphasized, and weaker in more individualistic societies. Additionally, growth mindset beliefs are more strongly related to personal well-being outcomes, such as emotional balance and life satisfaction, compared to occupational measures like job satisfaction. Finally, the domain of the mindset plays a role – beliefs about the malleability of teaching ability (as opposed to general intelligence) show stronger links to teacher well-being, especially in the workplace. These findings suggest that cultivating growth mindset beliefs may be particularly helpful for early-career teachers and in culturally supportive environments, with the greatest impact on personal emotional well-being.

Literature reviewed: Anderson et al., 2021; Barger et al., 2022; Elkheloufi & Fee Yean, 2022; Fathi & Soleimani, 2025; Frondozo et al., 2022; J. He et al., 2023; J. Kim et al., 2020; Kranjec & Tekavc, 2023; Lazarides & Schiepe-Tiska, 2022; E. O. Lee et al., 2023; L. Liu et al., 2023; Nalipay et al., 2019, 2021; Nicolosi et al., 2023; Shoshani, 2021; Tao et al., 2021; Tassell et al., 2020; Vettori et al., 2022; Xu & Wang, 2024; N. Yang, 2022; Zarrinabadi et al., 2023; Zeng et al., 2019; Zhaleh et al., 2018; Zilka et al., 2023.

5.6.1.1. Measure

Cultivate a growth mindset about your teaching ability by treating challenges as opportunities.

5.6.1.1.1. 3 Key Components

- **Reframe challenges with a 'yet' mindset**

  When setbacks occur, shift from 'I cannot do this' to 'I cannot do this yet.' View challenges as opportunities for learning by asking, 'What can I improve here?' to transform struggles into stepping stones for growth.

- **Reflect on past growth**

  Compare current challenges to situations you have successfully navigated before. Consider what strategies, efforts, or attitudes helped you succeed in the past. This practice reinforces the understanding that your abilities and skills grow through persistence and experience.

- **Set process goals, not just outcomes**

  Define success by what you practise and try (e.g. new strategies, effort, persistence) rather than only by results. This keeps motivation rooted in growth rather than in fixed benchmarks.

For Measure Dashboard, see Table 38.

5.6.1.2. Good-Practice Examples

5.6.1.2.1. Zambia: A Teacher's Transformation. A strong example of a teacher applying a growth mindset to their own development comes from a reflection shared through the Teach2030 programme in Zambia (Manda, 2021). The teacher described how they once held a fixed belief about intelligence, mentally labelling students as either 'intelligent' or 'dull', which shaped their expectations and responses. After completing a growth mindset course, they recognized this limiting outlook and deliberately shifted their approach. They now apply growth mindset principles in their own work – persevering when lessons are difficult, actively seeking and welcoming constructive feedback, and reframing others' success as inspiration rather than as a threat. By modelling this mindset, they not only strengthened their own resilience and sense of purpose but also fostered a more supportive, effort-focused classroom culture that improved learning outcomes for students.

Table 38. Measure Dashboard for Growth Mindset.

Dimension	Rating	Description
Impact	●●○ **Moderate**	Has a noticeable effect for some contexts or groups. Contributes meaningfully but not comprehensively
Quality of Evidence	●●● **High**	Strong, consistent evidence from rigorous research (e.g. meta-analyses, randomized controlled trials, longitudinal studies). Widely accepted in the field
Context Dependency	●●○ **Moderate**	Requires some adaptation but can function in several settings; effectiveness depends on moderately specific conditions (e.g. type of school)
Sustainability	●●○ **Moderate**	Some integration into structures or culture, but still somewhat dependent on leadership or budget
Teacher Voice	●●● **High**	Teachers co-design, adapt, and lead the initiative; their professional knowledge is central
Implementation Feasibility	●●○ **Moderate**	Requires some planning, adjustment, or collaboration. Feasible with committed leadership and moderate resource input

5.6.1.2.2. Tanzania: Collaborative Growth. A programme report from Tanzania described how teachers applied growth mindset principles in their own development. In a pilot project, 35 teachers attended monthly coaching sessions focused on growth mindset and deliberate practice (Teachers Acceleration Model and Growth Coaching, 2024). Participants reported that they were more willing to share and learn from each other. One teacher reflected, 'For me a growth mindset can be applied to our personal and professional life' (para. 3). Another teacher took a concrete instructional risk – she invited colleagues to teach alongside her in a large class. As she explained, 'As a result of what I've learnt through this program, my interaction with other teachers at my school has really improved' (para. 5), a change she made because of what she learned in the growth mindset training.

5.6.2. Experimentation

Experimentation in the workplace, understood as the deliberate testing of new ideas, methods, or routines to see what works best, has a clear and positive impact on well-being. When employees actively try out different approaches, they report lower levels of burnout and distress, along with higher job satisfaction. Structured initiatives that combine supportive leadership with greater control over one's work, or that encourage employees to build on their strengths and engage in job crafting, often result in meaningful improvements in both subjective and psychological well-being.

At the same time, even subtle, self-initiated changes, such as creating opportunities for flow or introducing small adjustments to the work environment, can reduce emotional exhaustion and boost positive mood.

What ties these approaches together is the way employees expand their job resources, increase their autonomy, and find greater meaning in their work. Context also matters – organizational culture, leadership style, and individual factors such as gender or job role shape how effective such experimentation will be.

Overall, workplaces in which employees are encouraged to experiment foster innovation and create conditions that sustain energy, engagement, and long-term well-being.

> Literature reviewed: Arnold, 2017; Dimotakis et al., 2010; Hu et al., 2017; Ilies et al., 2016; Koon & Ho, 2021; Krekel et al., 2019; Moen et al., 2016; Page & Vella-Brodrick, 2012; Rivkin et al., 2018; Tims et al., 2013.

5.6.2.1. Measure

Experiment with new approaches to your work.

5.6.2.1.1. 3 Key Components

- **Start small and stay curious**

  Choose one aspect of your work to experiment with at a time. Keep it manageable, like by trying a new way to start lessons, shifting group work, or testing a feedback method. Let curiosity be your guide.

- **Reflect and learn from outcomes**

  After each experiment, take a few minutes to note what worked, what did not, and what surprised you. Reflection helps you turn each attempt into a learning opportunity, boosting confidence and resilience.

- **Embrace flexibility and let go of perfection**

  View experimentation as practice, not performance. Give yourself permission to try, adjust, and sometimes fail without judgement. This mindset builds psychological safety and reduces stress while keeping your teaching dynamic.

For Measure Dashboard, see Table 39.

Table 39. Measure Dashboard for Experimentation.

Dimension	Rating	Description
Impact	●●○ **Moderate**	Has a noticeable effect for some contexts or groups. Contributes meaningfully but not comprehensively
Quality of Evidence	●●○ **Moderate**	Some research support, possibly from case studies or correlational data. Promising but not conclusive
Context Dependency	●●○ **Moderate**	Requires some adaptation but can function in several settings; effectiveness depends on moderately specific conditions (e.g. type of school)
Sustainability	●●○ **Moderate**	Some integration into structures or culture, but still somewhat dependent on leadership or budget
Teacher Voice	●●● **High**	Teachers co-design, adapt, and lead the initiative; their professional knowledge is central
Implementation Feasibility	●●○ **Moderate**	Requires some planning, adjustment, or collaboration. Feasible with committed leadership and moderate resource input

5.6.2.2. Good-Practice Example

5.6.2.2.1. Canada: Innovative Teaching Practices Enhance Teacher Well-Being. In a blog post, a Canadian teacher reported how she felt bored 5 years into her teaching career (Rawling, 2016). Seeking to reinvigorate her passion for teaching, she experimented with and delved into imaginative education, a pedagogical approach that integrates cognitive tools to make learning more engaging and meaningful. This shift allowed her to design lessons that were not only more captivating for students but also more fulfilling for her. By aligning her teaching with her personal interests and strengths, she found renewed enthusiasm for her work, leading to increased job satisfaction and a deeper connection with her students. This example illustrates how experimenting with new teaching strategies can positively impact teacher well-being, fostering a more dynamic and rewarding educational experience.

6

COMPLETE LIST OF MEASURES

This chapter brings together all the measures discussed throughout the book into a single, structured overview. To make it easy to use, the measures are organized according to their place within the nested doll system and follow the order in which they appear in the text. Fig. 6 provides a conceptual summary of the main priorities for supporting teacher well-being at each of the three levels.

In the following overview of measures (see Table 40), each entry includes the corresponding page number, so the more detailed discussion in the main text can be quickly located. In this way, the list serves as a navigational aid. Beyond orientation, the list can also be used as a practical tool. Three bubbles on the far left work as a checklist. The bubbles can be coloured in to

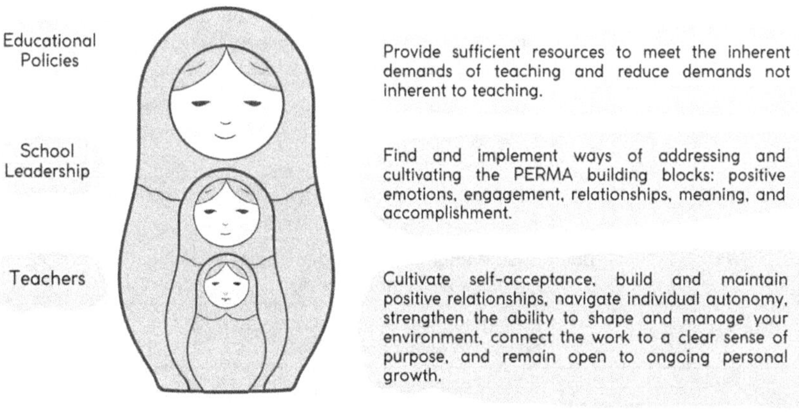

Fig. 6. Matryoshka Doll System for Fostering Teacher Well-Being. Figure Created by the Author.

mark the progress in implementing each measure. This transforms the list into a straightforward instrument for self-reflection, helping to recognize which measures have already been considered or implemented and which ones still need to be addressed.

Table 40. Overview of Measures and Checklist, Including Page Numbers for Additional Information.

Level of Implementation ●○○ Low ●●○ Moderate ●●● High	Nr.	Measure	More on page
		Educational Policies	
○○○	01	Implement sensible, context-sensitive class size limits.	20
○○○	02	Implement comprehensive workload regulations that reduce administrative burden, protect instructional time, and align teachers' responsibilities with their core professional roles.	23
○○○	03	Ensure the quality of teacher education and a focus on teacher well-being.	27
○○○	04	Guarantee competitive, fair, reliable, and context-appropriate teacher pay, particularly in low-income or crisis-affected settings.	29
○○○	05	Ensure meaningful, context-sensitive school autonomy, particularly in instructional decision-making and participatory governance.	31
○○○	06	Integrate consistent and meaningful appreciation into education policy, emphasizing recognition from students, parents, and school communities.	35
○○○	07	Make supportive leadership for teacher well-being a core requirement in school leadership standards and evaluation.	37
○○○	08	Integrate structured well-being programmes into all stages of the teaching profession.	39
○○○	09	Ensure equitable access to quality teaching materials and infrastructure.	42
○○○	10	Strengthen teacher voice and leadership in education policy and practice.	44
		School Leadership	
○○○	11	Establish and sustain a psychologically safe school environment.	50
○○○	12	Ensure that teachers regularly encounter and reflect on meaningful, affirming, and emotionally rewarding experiences.	53

Table 40. (*Continued*)

Level of Implementation ●○○ Low ●●○ Moderate ●●● High	Nr.	Measure	More on page
○○○	13	Build a culture of genuine appreciation and supportive communication.	55
○○○	14	Foster teaching autonomy by empowering decisions, easing constraints, and leading supportively.	57
○○○	15	Create an atmosphere where teachers feel encouraged to bring their personal interests into their work.	59
○○○	16	Foster conditions that enable teachers to experience flow in their daily work.	61
○○○	17	Empower teaching staff through sustained, responsive professional development that supports their well-being and professional purpose.	64
○○○	18	Build and sustain trust through transparent, supportive, and consistent leadership practices.	66
○○○	19	Cultivate a working culture of proactive, tailored social support.	69
○○○	20	Support positive student–teacher relationships.	71
○○○	21	Foster a culture of playfulness.	73
○○○	22	Promote shared educational goals and aligned values for your school.	75
○○○	23	Enable meaningful work through collective and individual job crafting.	78
○○○	24	Build and sustain collective efficacy.	80
○○○	25	Foster healthy achievement motivation.	82
		Teachers	
○○○	26	Practice self-compassion by treating yourself with the same kindness, patience, and understanding that you extend to others, especially when facing setbacks, mistakes, or stress.	87
○○○	27	Develop habits that actively build and sustain optimism in your daily work.	90
○○○	28	Strengthen emotional intelligence through reflective, mindful, and social–emotional practices.	93

(*Continued*)

Table 40. (*Continued*)

Level of Implementation ●○○ Low ●●○ Moderate ●●● High	Nr.	Measure	More on page
○○○	29	Actively seek out and engage with exemplary teaching and moral actions in others.	95
○○○	30	Foster high-quality connections in your school by intentionally creating small moments of care, trust, and support with colleagues throughout your day.	97
○○○	31	Set clear work–nonwork boundaries.	99
○○○	32	Prioritize restorative breaks during the school day.	102
○○○	33	Take control of your work by actively shaping your tasks, relationships, and approach to teaching to better fit your strengths and interests.	105
○○○	34	Set professional goals that focus on learning, growth, and continuous improvement rather than avoiding mistakes or comparing yourself to others.	107
○○○	35	Develop effective conflict and classroom management practices while recognizing and respecting your personal limits.	109
○○○	36	Perceive mentoring as a way to positively impact your own well-being while actively engaging in the development of the next generation of teachers.	112
○○○	37	Cultivate gratitude in your daily work practice.	114
○○○	38	Cultivate a growth mindset about your teaching ability by treating challenges as opportunities.	116
○○○	39	Experiment with new approaches to your work.	119

A PERSONAL NOTE

Everyone wants work that feels meaningful and fulfilling, and teachers are no exception. Yet teaching is a special profession – it has the power to shape entire generations. This book has gathered 39 research-based measures for strengthening teacher well-being across policy, school leadership, and individual practice, along with 55 examples of good practices from around the world. I believe these examples highlight that the presented measures are both relevant and feasible and that meaningful change is achievable. Yet, beneath the data lies a simple truth: People make education possible. As we reach the final pages, I want to speak directly to those involved.

To policymakers: You carry the responsibility of shaping the conditions under which learning and teaching unfold. We know the pressures you face: competing priorities, tight budgets, the need to show results quickly. This book is here to support you. Use the dashboards to identify the measures that are most impactful and sustainable. Share the book with colleagues, convene discussions across ministries and regions, and let it serve as common ground when political currents shift. Let the stories of teachers' voices guide you when choices are difficult. Your decisions can give teachers the stability and respect they deserve.

To school leaders: You stand close to the daily pulse of a school. This book is meant to help you care for your teams while caring for yourself. Bring it to your leadership team to reflect on and identify changes you can implement right away. Use the dashboards to compare measures and select those most suitable for your schools' needs to build the desired culture in the long term. At the same time, let the evidence help you advocate for larger policy or resource changes at council meetings or when speaking with district leaders and administrators.

To teachers: Every page of this book exists because of your persistence, creativity, and devotion to children. It is meant to help you identify what you can do to take charge of your own professional well-being and to spark ideas when it feels like there are no more options. Use the Measure Dashboards to pinpoint measures that you want to tackle next. Form peer groups around those that resonate, and pilot initiatives to show what is possible.

Finally, let the research and examples of good practice support your calls for fair conditions and respectful treatment, whether in union negotiations, staff committees, or one-on-one discussions with administrators.

This book now belongs to all of you. I hope you finish it not only with a clear overview of what supports teacher well-being but also with a sense of possibility. There is much that can be done and much that you can do to make teaching a sustainable, fulfilling profession.

ABOUT THE AUTHOR

Benjamin Dreer-Göthe is the Scientific Manager at the Erfurt School of Education, University of Erfurt, Germany, where he develops curricula, coordinates teacher education programmes, and conducts educational research. His research focuses on teacher well-being, examining concepts, influencing factors, interventions, and outcomes for preservice and in-service teachers. A sought-after expert, he serves as Associate Editor for *Frontiers in Education* and regularly reviews top publications in the field. He is also a member of the European Commission's Expert Group on Supportive Learning Environments and Well-being at School. In 2024, his research earned the Outstanding Paper Award from Emerald Publishing.

In 2025, he was nominated as a Highly Ranked Scholar by ScholarGPS in recognition of exceptional productivity, notable impact, and the quality of scholarly work in the speciality of well-being.

REFERENCES

Abbas, S., Shahzadi, A., Qaiser, N., & Islam, A. (2025). The impact of resilience and self-compassion on the psychological well-being of government school teachers in Sialkot. *ACADEMIA International Journal for Social Sciences*, *4*(1), 527–538. https://doi.org/10.63056/acad.004.01.0100

Abetang, M. A., Oguma, R. N., & Abetang, A. P. (2020). Mentoring and the difference it makes in teachers' work: A literature review. *European Journal of Education Studies*, *7*(6), 301–323. https://doi.org/10.46827/EJES.V7I6.3146

Acton, R., & Glasgow, P. (2015). Teacher wellbeing in neoliberal contexts: A review of the literature. *Australian Journal of Teacher Education*, *40*(8). https://doi.org/10.14221/ajte.2015v40n8.6

Akram, M., Munir, F., & Gilani, M. (2020). Relationship between emotional intelligence and psychological well-being of secondary school teachers. *Global Educational Studies Review*, *5*(4), 108–121. https://doi.org/10.31703/gesr.2020(v-iv).12

Albulescu, P., Macsinga, I., Rusu, A., Sulea, C., Bodnaru, A., & Tulbure, B. T. (2022). 'Give me a break!' A systematic review and meta-analysis on the efficacy of micro-breaks for increasing well-being and performance. *PLoS One*, *17*(8), e0272460. https://doi.org/10.1371/journal.pone.0272460

Alfes, K., Shantz, A., & Truss, C. (2012). The link between perceived practices, performance and well-being: The moderating effect of trust in the employer. *Human Resource Management Journal*, *22*(4), 409–427. https://doi.org/10.1111/1748-8583.12005

Algoe, S. B., & Haidt, J. (2009). Witnessing excellence in action: The 'other-praising' emotions of elevation, gratitude, and admiration. *The Journal of Positive Psychology*, *4*(2), 105–127. https://doi.org/10.1080/17439760802650519

AlHussaini, M. H., Amanat, I., & Munawar, N. (2024). Impact of professional development programs on early childhood teachers' well-being and classroom practices. *JECCE*, *8*(1), 76–93. https://doi.org/10.30971/jecce.v8i1.1982

Allen, K.-A., Grove, C., May, F. S., Gamble, N., Lai, R., & Saunders, J. M. (2024). Expressions of gratitude in education: An analysis of the #ThankYourTeacher campaign. *International Journal for Educational Integrity*, *20*(1), 13. https://doi.org/10.1007/s40979-024-00159-2

Alonso, C., Fernández-Salinero, S., & Topa, G. (2019). The impact of both individual and collaborative job crafting on Spanish teachers' well-being. *Education Sciences*, *9*(2), 74. https://doi.org/10.3390/educsci9020074

Amabile, T. M., Barsade, S. G., Mueller, J. S., & Staw, B. M. (2005). Affect and creativity at work. *Administrative Science Quarterly*, *50*(3), 367–403. https://doi.org/10.2189/asqu.2005.50.3.367

Ambition Institute. (2024, March 12). *Creating a strong school culture to improve behaviour and wellbeing*. https://www.ambition.org.uk/blog/creating-a-strong-school-culture-to-improve-behaviour-and-wellbeing/

Ames, C., & Archer, J. (1988). Achievement goals in the classroom: Students' learning strategies and motivation processes. *Journal of Educational Psychology*, *80*(3), 260–267. https://doi.org/10.1037/0022-0663.80.3.260

Anderson, R. C., Bousselot, T., Katz-Buoincontro, J., & Todd, J. (2021). Generating buoyancy in a sea of uncertainty: Teachers creativity and well-being during the covid-19 pandemic *Frontiers in Psychology*, *11*. https://doi.org/10.3389/fpsyg.2020.614774

Anderson, R. C., Katz-Buonincontro, J., Livie, M., Land, J., Beard, N., Bousselot, T., & Schuhe, G. (2022). Reinvigorating the desire to teach: Teacher professional development for creativity, agency, stress reduction, and wellbeing. *Frontiers in Education*, *7*. https://doi.org/10.3389/feduc.2022.848005

Arnold, K. A. (2017). Transformational leadership and employee psychological well-being: A review and directions for future research. *Journal of Occupational Health Psychology*, *22*(3), 381–393. https://doi.org/10.1037/ocp0000062

Arnold, K. A., Turner, N., Barling, J., Kelloway, E. K., & McKee, M. C. (2007). Transformational leadership and psychological well-being: The mediating role of meaningful work. *Journal of Occupational Health Psychology*, *12*(3), 193–203. https://doi.org/10.1037/1076-8998.12.3.193

Ashiedu, J. A., & Scott-Ladd, B. D. (2012). Understanding teacher attraction and retention drivers: Addressing teacher shortages. *Australian Journal of Teacher Education (Online)*, *37*(11), 23–41. http://ro.ecu.edu.au/ajte/vol37/iss11/2

Assaf, J., & Antoun, S. (2024). Impact of job satisfaction on teacher well-being and education quality. *Pedagogical Research*, *9*(3), em0204. https://doi.org/10.29333/pr/14437

Aulén, A.-M., Pakarinen, E., & Lerkkanen, M.-K. (2024). Teachers' job crafting to support their work-related well-being during the COVID-19 pandemic: A qualitative approach. *Teaching and Teacher Education*, *141*, 104492. https://doi.org/10.1016/j.tate.2024.104492

Australian Institute for Teaching and School Leadership. (2014). *Australian professional standard for principals and the leadership profiles.* https://tinyurl.com/2teudbe8

Avsec, A., Masnec, P., & Komidar, L. (2009). Personality traits and emotional intelligence as predictors of teachers' psychological well-being. *Horizons of Psychology*, *18*(3), 73–86.

Awwad-Tabry, S. (2024). Stretching boundaries: Unraveling teachers' challenges and strategies in cultivating self-compassion. *Journal of Psychiatry & Mental Disorders*, *95*(1), 1–7. https://doi.org/10.26420/jpsychiatrymentaldisord.2024.1074

Awwad-Tabry, S., & Levkovich, I. (2024). 'We felt so alone, but at least we felt it together': Self-compassion among teachers. *Psychology in the Schools*, *61*(12), 4465–4482. https://doi.org/10.1002/pits.23289

Baggett, M., Giambattista, L., Lobbestael, L., Pfeiffer, J., Madani, C., Modir, R., Zamora-Flyr, M. M., & Davidson, J. E. (2016). Exploring the human emotion of feeling cared for in the workplace. *Journal of Nursing Management*, *24*(6), 816–824. https://doi.org/10.1111/jonm.12388

Bajorek, Z., Gulliford, J., & Taskila, T. (2014). *Healthy teachers, higher marks? Establishing a link between teacher health and well-being, and student outcomes*. Education Support Partnership. https://rb.gy/wqoth7

Baker, M., & Ryan, J. (2021). Playful provocations and playful mindsets: Teacher learning and identity shifts through playful participatory research. *International Journal of Play*, *10*(1), 6–24. https://doi.org/10.1080/21594937.2021.1878770

Bakker, A. B., Demerouti, E., & Sanz-Vergel, A. (2023). Job demands–resources theory: Ten years later. *Annual Review of Organizational Psychology and Organizational Behavior*, *10*, 25–53. https://doi.org/10.1146/annurev-orgpsych-120920-053933

Bakker, A. B., Rodríguez-Muñoz, A., & Sanz Vergel, A. I. (2015). Modelling job crafting behaviours: Implications for work engagement. *Human Relations*, *69*(1), 169–189. https://doi.org/10.1177/0018726715581690

Bangs, J., R., & Frost, D. (2012). *Teacher self-efficacy, voice and leadership: Towards a policy framework for education international.* University of Cambridge. https://tinyurl.com/mvpfxpup

Bardach, L., & Klassen, R. M. (2021). Teacher motivation and student outcomes: Searching for the signal. *Educational Psychologist*, *56*(4), 283–297. https://doi.org/10.1080/00461520.2021.1991799

Barger, M., Xiong, Y., & Ferster, A. (2022). Identifying false growth mindsets in adults and implications for mathematics motivation. *Contemporary Educational Psychology*, *70*, 102079. https://doi.org/10.1016/j.cedpsych.2022.102079

Basom, M. R., & Frase, L. (2004). Creating optimal work environments: Exploring teacher flow experiences. *Mentoring & Tutoring: Partnership in Learning*, *12*(2), 241–258. https://doi.org/10.1080/1361126042000239965

Bass, B. M. (1995). Theory of transformational leadership redux. *The Leadership Quarterly*, *6*(4), 463–478. https://doi.org/10.1016/1048-9843(95)90021-7

Bassi, M., & Fave, A. D. (2012). Optimal experience among teachers: New insights into the work paradox. *The Journal of Psychology*, *146*(5), 533–557. https://doi.org/10.1080/00223980.2012.656156

Beames, J., Spanos, S., Roberts, A., McGillivray, L., Li, S., Newby, J., & Werner-Seidler, A. (2022). Intervention programs targeting the mental health, professional burnout, and/or wellbeing of school teachers: Systematic review and meta-analyses. *Educational Psychology Review*, *35*(26). https://doi.org/10.13140/RG.2.2.20489.31847

Beard, K. S., & Hoy, W. K. (2010). The nature, meaning, and measure of teacher flow in elementary schools: A test of rival hypotheses. *Educational Administration Quarterly*, *46*(3), 426–458. https://doi.org/10.1177/0013161x10375294

Becker, W. J., Belkin, L., & Tuskey, S. (2018). Killing me softly: Electronic communications monitoring and employee and spouse well-being. *Academy of Management Proceedings*, *2018*(1), 12574. https://doi.org/10.5465/ambpp.2018.121

Bell, K. (2024, September 17). *Sanity-saving classroom management tips every teacher needs.* Shake Up Learning. https://tinyurl.com/yw3zckmd

Belmonte, C., Estrella, J., & Eutsay, D. S. (2022). Social and emotional wellbeing of teachers and its impact on the teaching practice. *Journal of Education and Culture Studies*, *6*(1), 1. https://doi.org/10.22158/jecs.v6n1p1

Belyaeva, T. B., & Belyaeva, P. I. (2020). Personal qualities of teachers as factors of their psychological well-being. In S. A. Glebovich (Ed.), *Pedagogical education: History, present time, perspectives* (pp. 134–141). European Publisher. https://doi.org/10.15405/epsbs.2020.08.02.17

Benita, M., & Matos, L. (2021). Internalization of mastery goals: The differential effect of teachers' autonomy support and control. *Frontiers in Psychology*, *11*. https://doi.org/10.3389/fpsyg.2020.599303

Binnewies, C., Haun, V. C., Törk, J., Brauner, C., & Haun, S. (2020). The effects of boundary management strategies on employees' recovery and well-being. *Academy of Management Proceedings*, *2020*(1), 17134. https://doi.org/10.5465/ambpp.2020.17134

Binnewies, C., Sonnentag, S., & Mojza, E. J. (2009). Feeling recovered and thinking about the good sides of one's work. *Journal of Occupational Health Psychology*, *14*(3), 243–256. https://doi.org/10.1037/a0014933

Blasche, G., Pasalic, S., Bauböck, V.-M., Haluza, D., & Schoberberger, R. (2016). Effects of rest-break intention on rest-break frequency and work-related fatigue. *Human Factors: The Journal of the Human Factors and Ergonomics Society*, *59*(2), 289–298. https://doi.org/10.1177/0018720816671605

Blumenstock, J. E., Callen, M., Faikina, A., Fiorin, S., & Ghani, T. (2023). Strengthening fragile states: Evidence from mobile salary payments in Afghanistan. https://www.ifo.de/DocDL/cesifo1_wp10510.pdf

Bono, J. E., Glomb, T. M., Shen, W., Kim, E., & Koch, A. J. (2013). Building positive resources: Effects of positive events and positive reflection on work stress and health. *Academy of Management Journal*, *56*(6), 1601–1627. https://doi.org/10.5465/amj.2011.0272

Borralho, L., Candeias, A. A., de Jesus, S. N., & Viseu, J. (2025). Healthy school, healthy teachers: Mediating effect of optimism. *Frontiers in Psychology*, *16*. https://doi.org/10.3389/fpsyg.2025.1506161

Brady, J., & Wilson, E. (2020). Teacher wellbeing in England: Teacher responses to school-level initiatives. *Cambridge Journal of Education*, *51*(1), 45–63. https://doi.org/10.1080/0305764x.2020.1775789

Brough, P., & Pears, J. (2004). Evaluating the influence of the type of social support on job satisfaction and work related psychological well-being. *International Journal of Organisational Behaviour*, *8*(2), 472–485.

Brouwers, A., Evers, W. J. G., & Tomic, W. (2001). Self-efficacy in eliciting social support and burnout among secondary-school teachers. *Journal of Applied Social Psychology*, *31*(7), 1474–1491. https://doi.org/10.1111/j.1559-1816.2001.tb02683.x

Büchler, N., ter Hoeven, C. L., & van Zoonen, W. (2020). Understanding constant connectivity to work: How and for whom is constant connectivity related to employee well-being? *Information and Organization*, *30*(3), 100302. https://doi.org/10.1016/j.infoandorg.2020.100302

Bullough, R. V., Hall-Kenyon, K. M., & MacKay, K. L. (2012). Head start teacher well-being: Implications for policy and practice. *Early Childhood Education Journal*, *40*(6), 323–331. https://doi.org/10.1007/s10643-012-0535-8

Buonomo, I., Fiorilli, C., & Benevene, P. (2019). The impact of emotions and hedonic balance on teachers' self-efficacy: Testing the bouncing back effect of positive emotions. *Frontiers in Psychology*, *10*(1670). https://doi.org/10.3389/fpsyg.2019.01670

Buonomo, I., Fiorilli, C., & Benevene, P. (2020). Unravelling teacher job satisfaction: The contribution of collective efficacy and emotions towards professional role. *International Journal of Environmental Research and Public Health*, *17*(3), 736. https://doi.org/10.3390/ijerph17030736

Burić, I., & Frenzel, A. C. (2020). Teacher emotional labour, instructional strategies, and students' academic engagement: A multilevel analysis. *Teachers and Teaching*, *27*(5), 1–18. https://doi.org/10.1080/13540602.2020.1740194

Burić, I., & Moè, A. (2020). What makes teachers enthusiastic: The interplay of positive affect, self-efficacy and job satisfaction. *Teaching and Teacher Education*, *89*, 103008. https://doi.org/10.1016/j.tate.2019.103008

Butler, R. (2012). Striving to connect: Extending an achievement goal approach to teacher motivation to include relational goals for teaching. *Journal of Educational Psychology*, *104*(3), 726–742. https://doi.org/10.1037/a0028613

Canaslan-Akyar, B., & Sevimli-Celik, S. (2021). Playfulness of early childhood teachers and their views in supporting playfulness. *Education 50*(1), 1–15. https://doi.org/10.1080/03004279.2021.1921824

Cann, R. F., Riedel-Prabhakar, R., & Powell, D. (2020). A model of positive school leadership to improve teacher wellbeing. *International Journal of Applied Positive Psychology*, 6(2), 195–218. https://doi.org/10.1007/s41042-020-00045-5

Cann, R., Sinnema, C., Daly, A. J., & Rodway, J. (2024). A contextual approach to designing, implementing, and adapting a wellbeing program: A case study of the MARKERS wellbeing program for educators. *International Journal of Applied Positive Psychology*, *9*(1), 301–325. https://doi.org/10.1007/s41042-023-00123-4

Cano, S. L., Flores, B. B., Claeys, L., & Sass, D. A. (2017). Consequences of educator stress on turnover: The case of charter schools. In T. M. McIntyre, S. E. McIntyre, & D. J. Francis (Eds.), *Educator stress: An occupational health perspective* (pp. 127–156). Springer.

Caprara, G. V., Barbaranelli, C., Borgogni, L., & Steca, P. (2003). Efficacy beliefs as determinants of teachers' job satisfaction. *Journal of Educational Psychology*, *95*(4), 821–832. https://doi.org/10.1037/0022-0663.95.4.821

Caprara, G. V., Barbaranelli, C., Steca, P., & Malone, P. S. (2006). Teachers' self-efficacy beliefs as determinants of job satisfaction and students' academic achievement: A study at the school level. *Journal of School Psychology*, *44*, 473–490. https://doi.org/10.1016/j.jsp.2006.09.001

Carbonneau, N., Vallerand, R. J., Fernet, C., & Guay, F. (2008). The role of passion for teaching in intrapersonal and interpersonal outcomes. *Journal of Educational Psychology*, *100*(4), 977–987. https://doi.org/10.1037/a0012545

Carey, S., & Sutton, A. (2024). Early childhood teachers' emotional labour: The role of job and personal resources in protecting well-being. *Teaching and Teacher Education*, *148*, 104699. https://doi.org/10.1016/j.tate.2024.104699

Carlo, A., Michel, A., Chabanne, J.-C., Bucheton, D., Demougin, P., Herve, C., Kati, M., Leroux, G., Lichtenberger, Y., Melis, S., Pouchin, M., Probst, P., & Simon, D. (2013). *Study on policy measures to improve the attractiveness of the teaching profession in Europe (Research report EAC-2010-1391)*. European Commission. https://hal.archives-ouvertes.fr/hal-00922139

Carmeli, A., Brueller, D., & Dutton, J. E. (2008). Learning behaviours in the workplace: The role of high-quality interpersonal relationships and psychological safety. *Systems Research and Behavioral Science*, *26*(1), 81–98. https://doi.org/10.1002/sres.932

Carmeli, A., Reiter-Palmon, R., & Ziv, E. (2010). Inclusive leadership and employee involvement in creative tasks in the workplace: The mediating role of psychological safety. *Creativity Research Journal*, *22*(3), 250–260. https://doi.org/10.1080/10400419.2010.504654

Carpenter, D. M., Field, J. E., Tucker, E., & Ferguson, N. (2023). Evaluating teacher wellness professional development: A three-year study. *Educational Research: Theory and Practice*, *34*(1), 50–68.

Carroll, A., Forrest, K., Sanders-O'Connor, E., Flynn, L., Bower, J. M., Fynes-Clinton, S., York, A., & Ziaei, M. (2022). Teacher stress and burnout in Australia: Examining the role of intrapersonal and environmental factors. *Social Psychology of Education*, *25*(2–3), 441–469. https://doi.org/10.1007/s11218-022-09686-7

Castillo, I., Álvarez, O., Estevan, I., Queralt, A., & Molina-García, J. (2017). Passion for teaching, transformational leadership and burnout among physical education teachers. *Journal of Sport Psychology*, *26*(3), 57–61.

Cece, V., Guillet-Descas, E., & Lentillon-Kaestner, V. (2021). The longitudinal trajectories of teacher burnout and vigour across the scholar year: The predictive role of emotional intelligence. *Psychology in the Schools*, *59*(3), 589–606. https://doi.org/10.1002/pits.22633

Ceyanes, J. W., & Slater, R. (2005, April 15). *Does teacher trust in the principal influence teacher burnout* [Conference presentation]. American Educational Research Association (AREA) Annual Meeting, Montreal, Canada.

Chan, D. W. (2010). Gratitude, gratitude intervention and subjective well-being among Chinese school teachers in Hong Kong. *Educational Psychology*, *30*(2), 139–153. https://doi.org/10.1080/01443410903493934

Chan, D. W. (2011). Burnout and life satisfaction: Does gratitude intervention make a difference among Chinese school teachers in Hong Kong? *Educational Psychology*, *31*(7), 809–823. https://doi.org/10.1080/01443410.2011.608525

Cherkowski, S. (2018). Positive teacher leadership: Building mindsets and capacities to grow wellbeing. *International Journal of Teacher Leadership*, *9*(1), 1–16.

Chernikova, O. (2018). *What makes observational learning in teacher education effective? Evidence from a meta-analysis and an experimental study* [Doctoral dissertation, Ludwig-Maximilians-Universität, München]. https://t1p.de/5j3a2

Chhajer, R., & Dutta, T. (2021). Gratitude as a mechanism to form high-quality connections at work: Impact on job performance. *International Journal of Indian Culture and Business Management*, *22*(1), 1. https://doi.org/10.1504/ijicbm.2021.112613

Chi, H., Yeh, H., & Wu, S. F. (2014). How well-being mediates the relationship between social support and teaching effectiveness. *Journal of Education and Learning*, *3*(4), 117–130. https://doi.org/10.5539/jel.v3n4p117

Chowdhury, M. S. (2007). Enhancing motivation and work performance of the salespeople: The impact of supervisors' behavior. *The International Journal of Applied Management and Technology*, 6(1), 166–181.

Clark, S., & Newberry, M. (2019). Are we building preservice teacher self-efficacy? A large-scale study examining teacher education experiences. *Asia-Pacific Journal of Teacher Education*, *47*(1), 32–47. https://doi.org/10.1080/1359866X.2018.1497772

Clunies-Ross, P., Little, E., & Kienhuis, M. (2008). Self-reported and actual use of proactive and reactive classroom management strategies and their relationship with teacher stress and student behaviour. *Educational Psychology*, *28*(6), 693–710. https://doi.org/10.1080/01443410802206700

Collie, R. J. (2014). *Understanding teacher well-being and motivation: Measurement, theory, and change over time* [Doctoral dissertation, University of British Columbia]. https://doi.library.ubc.ca/10.14288/1.0165878

Collie, R. J. (2023). Teacher well-being and turnover intentions: Investigating the roles of job resources and job demands. *British Journal of Educational Psychology*, *93*(3), 712–726. https://doi.org/10.1111/bjep.12587

Collie, R. J., Perry, N. E., & Martin, A. J. (2017). School context and educational system factors impacting educator stress. In T. M. McIntyre, S. E. McIntyre, & D. J. Francis (Eds.), *Educator stress: An occupational health perspective* (pp. 3–22). Springer.

Collie, R. J., Shapka, J. D., & Perry, N. E. (2012). School climate and social–emotional learning: Predicting teacher stress, job satisfaction, and teaching efficacy. *Journal of Educational Psychology*, *104*(4), 1189–1204. https://doi.org/10.1037/a0029356

Collie, R. J., Shapka, J. D., Perry, N. E., & Martin, A. J. (2016). Teachers' psychological functioning in the workplace: Exploring the roles of contextual beliefs, need satisfaction, and personal characteristics. *Journal of Educational Psychology*, *108*(6), 788–799. https://doi.org/10.1037/edu0000088

Compen, B., De Witte, K., & Schelfhout, W. (2020). The impact of teacher engagement in an interactive webinar series on the effectiveness of financial literacy education. *British Journal of Educational Technology*, *52*(1), 411–425. https://doi.org/10.1111/bjet.13013

Corbin, C. M., Alamos, P., Lowenstein, A. E., Downer, J. T., & Brown, J. L. (2019). The role of teacher–student relationships in predicting teachers' personal accomplishment and emotional exhaustion. *Journal of School Psychology*, *77*, 1–12. https://doi.org/10.1016/j.jsp.2019.10.001

Corrigan, D., & Loughran, J. (2008). *Mentoring for the teaching profession: Snapshots of practice* [Conference proceeding]. British Educational Research Association Annual Conference, Edinburgh. http://www.beraconference.co.uk/2008/index.html

Costantini, A., & Sartori, R. (2018). The intertwined relationship between job crafting, work-related positive emotions, and work engagement. Evidence from a positive psychology intervention study. *The Open Psychology Journal*, *11*(1), 210–221. https://doi.org/10.2174/1874350101811010210

Crissman, J. (2006, January 01). *The design and utilization of effective worked examples: A meta-analysis* [Doctoral Dissertation, University of Nebraska]. https://digitalcommons.unl.edu/cgi/viewcontent.cgi?article=11198&context=dissertations

Cronin, S. (2018, October 25). *Hacking leadership with passion projects.* The Shift Blog. https://hdsb-theshift.blogspot.com/2018/10/hacking-leadership-with-passion-projects.html

Crosswell, L., & Elliott, R. (2004, n.d.). *Committed teachers, passionate teachers: The dimension of passion associated with teacher commitment and engagement* [Paper presentation]. Australian Association for Research in Education (AARE) Annual Conference, Melbourne.

Cuevas, R., Ntoumanis, N., Fernandez-Bustos, J. G., & Bartholomew, K. (2018). Does teacher evaluation based on student performance predict motivation, well-being, and ill-being? *Journal of School Psychology*, *68*, 154–162. https://doi.org/10.1016/j.jsp.2018.03.005

Cuyvers, K., Weerd, G. D., Dupont, S. F., Mols, S., & Nuytten, C. (2011). *Well-being at school.* CELE Exchange, Centre for Effective Learning Environments. https://doi.org/10.1787/5kg0lkzc81vc-en

Cvenkel, N. R. (2018). Employee well-being at work: Insights for business leaders and corporate social responsibility. In S. Seifi & D. Crowther (Eds.), *Developments in corporate governance and responsibility* (pp. 71–90). Emerald Publishing. https://doi.org/10.1108/s2043-052320180000014004

D'Amico, A., Geraci, A., & Tarantino, C. (2020). The relationship between perceived emotional intelligence, work engagement, job satisfaction, and burnout in Italian school teachers. *Psihologijske teme*, *29*(1), 63–84. https://doi.org/10.31820/pt.29.1.4

Dababneh, A. J., Swanson, N., & Shell, R. L. (2001). Impact of added rest breaks on the productivity and well being of workers. *Ergonomics*, *44*(2), 164–174. https://doi.org/10.1080/00140130121538

Dahal, G. (2023). Collaborative mentoring for in-service teachers' well-being in the Nepalese context. *Journal of NELTA Gandaki*, *6*(1–2), 89–97. https://doi.org/10.3126/jong.v6i1-2.59715

Daniel, S., & Sonnentag, S. (2014). Work to non-work enrichment: The mediating roles of positive affect and positive work reflection. *Work & Stress*, *28*(1), 49–66. https://doi.org/10.1080/02678373.2013.872706

Dave, D. J., McClure, L. A., Rojas, S. R., De Lavalette, O., & Lee, D. J. (2020). Impact of mindfulness training on the well-being of educators. *The Journal of Alternative and Complementary Medicine*, *26*(7), 645–651. https://doi.org/10.1089/acm.2019.0451

Day, C., & Kington, A. (2008). Identity, well-being and effectiveness: the emotional contexts of teaching. *Pedagogy, Culture & Society*, *16*(1), 7–23. https://doi.org/10.1080/14681360701877743

Demerouti, E., Bakker, A. B., Nachreiner, F., & Schaufeli, W. B. (2001). The job demands-resources model of burnout. *The Journal of Applied Psychology*, *86*(3), 499–512. http://dx.doi.org/10.1037/0021-9010.86.3.499

Department for Education. (2023, November 1). *Be that teacher*. Australian Government. https://www.education.gov.au/newsroom/articles/be-teacher-national-campaign

Department for Education. (2024). *Initial teacher training (ITT): Core content framework*. UK Government. https://www.gov.uk/government/publications/initial-teacher-training-itt-core-content-framework

Department for Education. (2025, May 23). *More teachers to benefit from flexible working*. UK Government. https://www.gov.uk/government/news/more-teachers-to-benefit-from-flexible-working

Derickson, R., Fishman, J., Osatuke, K., Teclaw, R., & Ramsel, D. (2015). Psychological safety and error reporting within veterans health administration hospitals. *Journal of Patient Safety*, *11*(1), 60–66. https://doi.org/10.1097/pts.0000000000000082

Dias, N., & Arachchige, B. (2014). Using a double-edged sword: Emotional labour and the well-being of teachers in a national school in Sri Lanka. Proceedings of the 11th International Conference on Business Management.

Dierenfeld, C. M. (2024). Unlocking fun: Accessing play to enhance secondary teachers' well-being. *Teaching and Teacher Education*, *142*, 104523. https://doi.org/10.1016/j.tate.2024.104523

Dimotakis, N., Scott, B. A., & Koopman, J. (2010). An experience sampling investigation of workplace interactions, affective states, and employee well-being. *Journal of Organizational Behavior*, *32*(4), 572–588. https://doi.org/10.1002/job.722

Ding, K., & Rohlfs, C. (2020). Ursachenzuschreibungen eigener Unterrichts(miss)erfolge Lehramtsstudierender und ihr Zusammenhang mit einer Veränderung der Selbstwirksamkeitserwartung: Eine Mixed-Methods-Studie [Attributions of preservice teachers' own instructional (mis)successes and their relation to changes in self-efficacy beliefs: A mixed-methods study]. *BzL - Beiträge zur Lehrerinnen- und Lehrerbildung*, *38*(2), 274–291. https://doi.org/10.36950/bzl.38.2.2020.9306

Dreer, B. (2020). Positive psychological interventions for teachers: A randomised placebo-controlled field experiment investigating the effects of workplace-related positive activities. *International Journal of Applied Positive Psychology*, *5*, 77–97. https://doi.org/10.1007/s41042-020-00027-7

Dreer, B. (2022). Teacher well-being: Investigating the contributions of school climate and job crafting. *Cogent Education*, *9*(1). https://doi.org/10.1080/2331186X.2022.2044583

Dreer, B. (2023a). On the outcomes of teacher wellbeing: A systematic review of research. *Frontiers in Psychology*, *14*. https://doi.org/10.3389/fpsyg.2023.1205179

Dreer, B. (2023b). Witnessing well-being in action: Observing teacher well-being during field experiences predicts student teacher well-being. *Frontiers in Education*, *8*. https://doi.org/10.3389/feduc.2023.967905

Dreer, B., Dietrich, J., & Kracke, B. (2017). From in-service teacher development to school improvement: Factors of learning transfer in teacher education. *Teacher Development*, *21*(2), 208–224. https://doi.org/10.1080/13664530.2016.1224774

Dreer, B., & Gouasé, N. (2021). Interventions fostering well-being of schoolteachers: A review of research. *Oxford Review of Education*, *48*(5), 587–605. https://doi.org/10.1080/03054985.2021.2002290

Dreer, B., & Kracke, B. (2021). Lehrer*innen im Corona-Lockdown 2020 – Umgang mit der Distanzbetreuung im Spannungsfeld von Anforderungen und Ressourcen [Teachers* in corona-lockdown 2020: Dealing with distance teaching based on demands and resources]. In C. Reintjes, R. Porsch, & G. im Brahm (Eds.), *Das Bildungssystem in Zeiten der Krise. Empirische Befunde, Konsequenzen und Potentiale für das Lehren und Lernen [The education system in times of crisis. Empirical findings, consequences and potentials for teaching and learning]* (pp. 54–62). Waxmann.

Dreer-Goethe, B. (2023). Well-being and mentoring in pre-service teacher education: An integrative literature review. *International Journal of Mentoring and Coaching in Education*, 12(4), 336–349. https://doi.org/10.1108/ijmce-09-2022-0073

Dreer-Goethe, B. (2025a). Embracing variety: How different perceptions of teacher wellbeing can contribute to enhanced work experiences. *Frontiers in Education*, *10*. https://doi.org/10.3389/feduc.2025.1535497

Dreer-Goethe, B. (2025b). How appreciation predicts teachers' job satisfaction, emotional exhaustion, and quitting intentions. *Educational Studies*. https://doi.org/10.1080/03055698.2025.2511915

Dreer-Goethe, B. (2025c). The impact of mentor support and high-quality connections on student teachers' psychological safety and engagement during practicum. *Frontiers in Education*, *10*. https://doi.org/10.3389/feduc.2025.1499749

Dreer-Goethe, B. (2025d). The effects of emotional labour on well-being among shy student teachers. *International Journal of Educational Research Open*, *9*. https://doi.org/10.1016/j.ijedro.2025.100526

Dreer-Goethe, B. (2025e). *Moments that matter: How critical incidents shape the well-being of student teachers during their practicum*. [Manuscript submitted for publication].

Dutton, J. E. (2017). Let's bet on high quality connecting as a path for fostering well-being at work. In M. A. White, G. R. Slemp, & A. S. Murray (Eds.),

Future directions in well-being: Education, organizations and policy (pp. 111–115). Springer International Publishing. https://doi.org/10.1007/978-3-319-56889-8_20

Dutton, J. E., & Heaphy, E. (2005). *Embodying social interactions: Integrating physiology into the study of connections and relationships at work*. University of Michigan. https://deepblue.lib.umich.edu/bitstream/handle/2027.42/39172/1013.pdf?sequence=1&isAllowed=y

Dutton, J. E., & Heaphy, E. D. (2003). The power of high-quality connections. *Positive Organizational Scholarship: Foundations of a New Discipline*, *3*, 263–278.

Dutton, J. E., & Ragins, B. R. (2007). Moving forward: Positive relationships at work as a research frontier. In J. E. Dutton & B. R. Ragins (Eds.), *Exploring positive relationships at work: Building a theoretical and research foundation* (pp. 387–400). Lawrence Erlbaum Associates Publishers.

Dye, L., Burke, M. G., & Wolf, C. (2019). Teaching mindfulness for the self-care and well-being of counselors-in-training. *Journal of Creativity in Mental Health*, *15*(2), 140–153. https://doi.org/10.1080/15401383.2019.1642171

Dysvik, A., & Kuvaas, B. (2012). Intrinsic and extrinsic motivation as predictors of work effort: The moderating role of achievement goals. *British Journal of Social Psychology*, *52*(3), 412–430. https://doi.org/10.1111/j.2044-8309.2011.02090.x

Eder, F., Dämon, K., & Hörl, G. (2011). Das „Autonomie-Paritäts-Muster": Vorberuflich erlerntes Stereotyp, Bewältigungsstrategie oder Ergebnis der beruflichen Sozialisation? [The "autonomy–parity pattern": A pre-vocationally acquired stereotype, coping strategy, or result of professional socialization?]. *Zeitschrift für Bildungsforschung*, *1*(3), 199–217. https://doi.org/10.1007/s35834-011-0021-1

Education Scotland. (2025). *Professional learning: Health and wellbeing webinar series*. https://tinyurl.com/2rmhem3a

Elkheloufi, A., & Fee Yean, T. (2022). The mediating role of positive emotions in growth mindsets and work engagement relationship among Algerian academics. *Journal of Positive School Psychology*, 6(3), 1571–1586.

Eloff, I., & Dittrich, A.-K. (2021). Understanding general pedagogical knowledge influences on sustainable teacher well-being: A qualitative exploratory study. *Journal of Psychology in Africa*, *31*(5), 464–469. https://doi.org/10.1080/14330237.2021.1978166

Essex Research School. (2025, March 17). *Spotlights on success: How teacher-led PD brightens schools*. https://researchschool.org.uk/essex/news/spotlights-on-success-how-teacher-led-pd-brightens-schools

Eun, B., & Heining-Boynton, A. L. (2007). Impact of an English-as-a-second-language professional development program. *The Journal of Educational Research*, *101*(1), 36–49. https://doi.org/10.3200/joer.101.1.36-49

Even-Zahav, A., Widder, M., & Hazzan, O. (2022). From teacher professional development to teacher personal-professional growth: The case of expert STEM teachers. *Teacher Development*, *26*(3), 299–316. https://doi.org/10.1080/13664530.2022.2052947

Eysel-Gosepath, K., Daut, T., Pinger, A., Lehmacher, W., & Erren, T. (2013). Technical briefs. *Noise & Vibration Worldwide*, *44*(5), 23–28. https://doi.org/10.1260/0957-4565.44.5.23

Falk, D., Shephard, D., & Mendenhall, M. E. D. (2022). 'I always take their problem as mine': Understanding the relationship between teacher–student relationships and teacher well-being in crisis contexts. *International Journal of Educational Development*, *95*, 102670. https://doi.org/10.1016/j.ijedudev.2022.102670

Farley, A. N., & Chamberlain, L. M. (2021). The teachers are not alright: A call for research and policy on teacher stress and well-being. *The New Educator*, *17*(3), 305–323. https://doi.org/10.1080/1547688x.2021.1939918

Farley, A., Kennedy-Behr, A., & Brown, T. (2021). An investigation into the relationship between playfulness and well-being in Australian adults: An exploratory study. *Occupational Therapy Journal of Research*, *41*(1), 56–64. https://doi.org/10.1177/1539449220945311

Fathi, J., & Soleimani, H. (2025). Enhancing well-being: Exploring the influence of teacher growth mindset and grit among EFL instructors in Iran. *Language Related Research*, *16*(1), 219–247. https://doi.org/10.48311/lrr.16.1.219

Fauteux, M. (2018, December 29). *Building school culture with gratitude*. Getting Smart. https://www.gettingsmart.com/2018/12/29/building-school-culture-with-gratitude/

Feng, X., & Han, P. (2023). Today, tomorrow, and then forever: Exploring how workflow experience is sustained from a work–home perspective. *Journal of Management & Organization*, *30*(5), 1585–1606. https://doi.org/10.1017/jmo.2023.61

Fernández-Berrocal, P., Gutiérrez-Cobo, M. J., Rodriguez-Corrales, J., & Cabello, R. (2017). Teachers' affective well-being and teaching experience: The protective role of perceived emotional intelligence. *Frontiers in Psychology*, *8*. https://doi.org/10.3389/fpsyg.2017.02227

Fernet, C., Lavigne, G. L., Vallerand, R. J., & Austin, S. (2014). Fired up with passion: Investigating how job autonomy and passion predict burnout at career start in teachers. *Work & Stress*, *28*(3), 270–288. https://doi.org/10.1080/02678373.2014.935524

Fiorilli, C., Benevene, P., De Stasio, S., Buonomo, I., Romano, L., Pepe, A., & Addimando, L. (2019). Teachers' burnout: The role of trait emotional intelligence and social support. *Frontiers in Psychology*, *10*. https://doi.org/10.3389/fpsyg.2019.02743

Fogelgarn, R., & Burns, E. A. (2020). What constrains passionate teaching? A heuristic exploration. *Issues in Educational Research*, *30*(2), 493–511.

Ford, T. G., Olsen, J., Khojasteh, J., Ware, J., & Urick, A. (2019). The effects of leader support for teacher psychological needs on teacher burnout, commitment, and intent to leave. *Journal of Educational Administration*, *57*(6), 615–634. https://doi.org/10.1108/jea-09-2018-0185

Forster, M., Kuhbandner, C., & Hilbert, S. (2022). Teacher well-being: teachers' goals and emotions for students showing undesirable behaviors count more than that for students showing desirable behaviors. *Frontiers in Psychology*, *13*. https://doi.org/10.3389/fpsyg.2022.842231

Fouché, E., Rothmann, S., & van der Vyver, C. (2017). Antecedents and outcomes of meaningful work among school teachers. *SA Journal of Industrial Psychology*, *43*, 1–10. http://www.scielo.org.za/scielo.php?script=sci_arttext&pid=S2071-07632017000100005&nrm=iso

Fowler, S., Gabriel, F., & Leonard, S. N. (2022). Exploring the effect of teacher ontological and epistemic cognition on engagement with professional development. *Professional Development in Education*, *51*(2), 319–335. https://doi.org/10.1080/19415257.2022.2131600

Fox, H. B., Tuckwiller, E. D., Kutscher, E. L., & Walter, H. L. (2020). What makes teachers well? *Journal of Interdisciplinary Studies in Education*, *9*(2), 233–257. https://doi.org/10.32674/jise.v9i2.2170

Fox, K. E., Johnson, S. T., Berkman, L. F., Sianoja, M., Soh, Y., Kubzansky, L. D., & Kelly, E. L. (2021). Organisational- and group-level workplace interventions and their effect on multiple domains of worker well-being:

A systematic review. *Work & Stress*, *36*(1), 30–59. https://doi.org/10.1080/02678373.2021.1969476

Fradkin-Hayslip, A. (2021). Teacher autonomy, motivation, and job satisfaction: Perceptions of elementary school teachers according to self-determination theory. *İlköğretim Online*, *20*(2).

Fredrickson, B. L. (2001). The role of positive emotions in positive psychology: The broaden-and-build-theory of positive emotions *American Psychologist*, *56*, 218–226. https://doi.org/10.1037//0003-066x.56.3.218

French, J. R. P. (1953). Experiments in field settings. In L. Festinger & D. Katz (Eds.), *Research methods in the behavioral sciences* (pp. 98–135). Dryden Press.

French, N. (1993). Elementary teacher stress and class size. *Journal of Research & Development in Education*, 26(2), 66–73.

Frenzel, A. C. (2014). Teacher emotions. In A. Linnenbrink-Garcia & R. Pekrun (Eds.), *International handbook of emotions in education* (pp. 494–519). Routledge.

Frondozo, C. E., King, R. B., Nalipay, M. J. N., & Mordeno, I. G. (2022). Mindsets matter for teachers, too: Growth mindset about teaching ability predicts teachers' enjoyment and engagement. *Current Psychology*, *41*(8), 5030–5033. https://doi.org/10.1007/s12144-020-01008-4

Fundacion Chile. (2025). *Teacher support in a diverse classroom: Portal educarchile*. https://fch.cl/en/initiative/learning-for-the-future/

Gardner, D. M., & Prasad, J. J. (2022). The consequences of being myself: Understanding authenticity and psychological safety for LGB employees. *Journal of Occupational and Organizational Psychology*, *95*(4), 788–797. https://doi.org/10.1111/joop.12399

Garrick, A., Mak, A. S., Cathcart, S., Winwood, P. C., Bakker, A. B., & Lushington, K. (2014). Psychosocial safety climate moderating the effects of daily job demands and recovery on fatigue and work engagement. *Journal of Occupational and Organizational Psychology*, *87*(4), 694–714. https://doi.org/10.1111/joop.12069

Gerlach, R., & Gockel, C. (2017). We belong together: Belonging to the principal's in-group protects teachers from the negative effects of task conflict on psychological safety. *School Leadership & Management*, *38*(3), 302–322. https://doi.org/10.1080/13632434.2017.1407307

Ghamrawi, N., Naccache, H., & Shal, T. (2023). Teacher leadership and teacher wellbeing: Any relationship? *International Journal of Educational Research*, *122*, 102261. https://doi.org/10.1016/j.ijer.2023.102261

Ghasemi, F. (2022). The effects of dysfunctional workplace behavior on teacher emotional exhaustion: A moderated mediation model of perceived social support and anxiety. *Psychological Reports*, *127*(5), 2526–2551. https://doi.org/10.1177/00332941221146699

Gibbons, S., & Newberry, M. (2022). Exploring self-compassion as a means of emotion regulation in teaching. *Teacher Development*, *27*(1), 19–35. https://doi.org/10.1080/13664530.2022.2149613

Gillet, N., Lafrenière, M. A. K., Vallerand, R. J., Huart, I., & Fouquereau, E. (2012). The effects of autonomous and controlled regulation of performance-app roach goals on well-being: A process model. *British Journal of Social Psychology*, *53*(1), 154–174. https://doi.org/10.1111/bjso.12018

Glavin, P., & Schieman, S. (2025). The job satisfaction paradox: Pluralistic ignorance and the myth of the 'unhappy worker'. *Social Psychology Quarterly*, *88*(1), 22–44. https://doi.org/10.1177/01902725241253252

Gonzalez, J. A. (2019, May 3). *The faculty and staff survey: A tool for leadership growth*. Cult of Pedagogy. https://www.cultofpedagogy.com/faculty-staff-survey-form/

Good, A. G., Fox Barocas, S., Chávez-Moreno, L. C., Feldman, R., & Canela, C. (2017). A seat at the table: How the work of teaching impacts teachers as policy agents. *Peabody Journal of Education*, 92(4), 505–520. https://doi.org/10.1080/0161956x.2017.1349490

Grajeda, E. M. (2024, November 20). *How mentorship has kept me in the classroom*. EdSurge. https://tinyurl.com/4ya65fux

Greene, M. (1984). Teacher education against the darkness. *Focus on Learning*, *10*(2), 8–13.

Greenglass, E. R., Burke, R. J., & Konarski, R. (1997). The impact of social support on the development of burnout in teachers: Examination of a model. *Work & Stress*, *11*(3), 267–278. https://doi.org/10.1080/02678379708256840

Greenglass, E., Fiksenbaum, L., & Burke, R. J. (1996). Components of social support, buffering effects and burnout: Implications for psychological functioning. *Anxiety, Stress & Coping*, 9(3), 185–197. https://doi.org/10.1080/10615809608249401

Gregersen, S., Vincent-Höper, S., & Nienhaus, A. (2014). Health-relevant leadership behaviour: A comparison of leadership constructs. *German Journal of Human Resource Management: Zeitschrift für Personalforschung*, *28*(1–2), 117–138. https://doi.org/10.1177/239700221402800107

Griffith, J., Steptoe, A., & Cropley, M. (1999). An investigation of coping strategies associated with job stress in teachers. *British Journal of Educational Psychology*, *69*(4), 517–531. https://doi.org/10.1348/000709999157879

Guidetti, G., Viotti, S., Bruno, A., & Converso, D. (2018). Teachers' work ability: A study of relationships between collective efficacy and self-efficacy beliefs. *Psychology Research and Behavior Management*, *11*, 197–206. https://doi.org/10.2147/prbm.s157850

Hafenbrack, A. C., & Vohs, K. D. (2018). Mindfulness meditation impairs task motivation but not performance. *Organizational Behavior and Human Decision Processes*, *147*, 1–15. https://doi.org/10.1016/j.obhdp.2018.05.001

Hahn, V. C., & Dormann, C. (2013). The role of partners and children for employees' psychological detachment from work and well-being. *Journal of Applied Psychology*, *98*(1), 26–36. https://doi.org/10.1037/a0030650

Hakanen, J. J., Seppälä, P., & Peeters, M. C. W. (2017). High job demands, still engaged and not burned out? The role of job crafting. *International Journal of Behavioral Medicine*, *24*(4), 619–627. https://doi.org/10.1007/s12529-017-9638-3

Haldimann, M., Morinaj, J., & Hascher, T. (2023). The role of dyadic teacher–student relationships for primary school teachers' well-being. *International Journal of Environmental Research and Public Health*, *20*(5), 4053. https://doi.org/10.3390/ijerph20054053

Hanushek, E. A., Link, S., & Woessmann, L. (2012). Does school autonomy make sense everywhere? Panel estimates from PISA. *SSRN Electronic Journal*. https://doi.org/10.2139/ssrn.2017307

Harding, S., Morris, R., Gunnell, D., Ford, T., Hollingworth, W., Tilling, K., Evans, R., Bell, S., Grey, J., Brockman, R., Campbell, R., Araya, R., Murphy, S., & Kidger, J. (2019). Is teachers' mental health and wellbeing associated with students' mental health and wellbeing? *Journal of Affective Disorders*, *242*, 180–187. https://doi.org/10.1016/j.jad.2018.08.080

Hascher, T., & Waber, J. (2021). Teacher well-being: A systematic review of the research literature from the year 2000–2019. *Educational Research Review*, *34*, 100411. https://doi.org/10.1016/j.edurev.2021.100411

Hasnain, S. (2023). A review on the well-being of school teachers. *International Journal of Multidisciplinary Research and Growth Evaluation*, *4*(4), 519–523. https://doi.org/10.54660/.ijmrge.2023.4.4.519-523

Haworth, J. T., Jarman, M., & Lee, S. (1997). Positive psychological states in the daily life of a sample of working women. *Journal of Applied Social Psychology*, *27*(4), 345–370. https://doi.org/10.1111/j.1559-1816.1997.tb00636.x

He, Y., & Bagwell, D. (2021). Supporting teachers working with English learners: Engagement and impact of a professional development program. *TESOL Journal*, *13*(1). https://doi.org/10.1002/tesj.632

He, J., Iskhar, S., Yang, Y., & Aisuluu, M. (2023). Exploring the relationship between teacher growth mindset, grit, mindfulness, and EFL teachers' well-being. *Frontiers in Psychology*, *14*. https://doi.org/10.3389/fpsyg.2023.1241335

Heidemeier, H., & Wiese, B. S. (2014). Achievement goals and autonomy: How person–context interactions predict effective functioning and well-being during a career transition. *Journal of Occupational Health Psychology*, *19*(1), 18–31. https://doi.org/10.1037/a0034929

Henning, R. A., Jacques, P., Kissel, G. V., Sullivan, A. B., & Alteras-Webb, S. M. (1997). Frequent short rest breaks from computer work: Effects on productivity and well-being at two field sites. *Ergonomics*, *40*(1), 78–91. https://doi.org/10.1080/001401397188396

Herman, K. C., Hickmon-Rosa, J., & Reinke, W. M. (2017). Empirically derived profiles of teacher stress, burnout, self-efficacy, and coping and associated student outcomes. *Journal of Positive Behavior Interventions*, *20*(2), 90–100. https://doi.org/10.1177/1098300717732066

Herrera, C., Torres-Vallejos, J., Martínez-Líbano, J., Rubio, A., Céspedes, C., Oyanedel, J. C., Acuña, E., & Pedraza, D. (2022). Perceived collective school efficacy mediates the organizational justice effect in teachers' subjective well-being. *International Journal of Environmental Research and Public Health*, *19*(17), 10963. https://doi.org/10.3390/ijerph191710963

Hickman, A. (2025, May 29). *When your classroom is your bedroom: Setting boundaries (before burnout) for remote teachers*. Been Remote. https://www.beenremote.com/remote-work/boundaries-as-a-teacher#:~:text=,negotiable

Himalayan Trust UK. (2025, March 1). *From silence to smiles: Transforming classrooms in Nepal*. https://tinyurl.com/45j78mx7

Hojo, M. (2021). Association between student-teacher ratio and teachers' working hours and workload stress: Evidence from a nationwide survey in Japan. *BMC Public Health*, *21*(1), 1635. https://doi.org/10.1186/s12889-021-11677-w

Hollweck, T. (2019). 'I love this stuff!': A Canadian case study of mentor–coach well-being. *International Journal of Mentoring and Coaching in Education*, *8*(4), 325–344. https://doi.org/10.1108/ijmce-02-2019-0036

Hoobler, J. M., Rospenda, K. M., Lemmon, G., & Rosa, J. A. (2010). A within-subject longitudinal study of the effects of positive job experiences and generalized workplace harassment on well-being. *Journal of Occupational Health Psychology*, *15*(4), 434–451. https://doi.org/10.1037/a0021000

Howells, K. (2014). An exploration of the role of gratitude in enhancing teacher–student relationships. *Teaching and Teacher Education*, *42*, 58–67. https://doi.org/10.1016/j.tate.2014.04.004

Howells, K. D. (2024). *How can we practice gratitude in education?* Grateful Living. https://tinyurl.com/y5r6sxzw

Hu, X., Zhan, Y., Yao, X., & Garden, R. (2017). Picture this: A field experiment of the influence of subtle affective stimuli on employee well-being and performance. *Journal of Organizational Behavior*, *38*(6), 895–916. https://doi.org/10.1002/job.2177

Huang, S., Yin, H., & Lv, L. (2019). Job characteristics and teacher well-being: The mediation of teacher self-monitoring and teacher self-efficacy. *Educational Psychology*, *39*(3), 313–331. https://doi.org/10.1080/01443410.2018.1543855

Hue, M., & Lau, N. (2015). Promoting well-being and preventing burnout in teacher education: A pilot study of a mindfulness-based programme for pre-service teachers in Hong Kong. *Teacher Development*, *19*(3), 381–401. https://doi.org/10.1080/13664530.2015.1049748

Hunter, E. M., & Wu, C. (2016). Give me a better break: Choosing workday break activities to maximize resource recovery. *Journal of Applied Psychology*, *101*(2), 302–311. https://doi.org/10.1037/apl0000045

Ilies, R., Bono, J. E., & Bakker, A. B. (2024). Crafting well-being: Employees can enhance their own well-being by savoring, reflecting upon, and capitalizing on positive work experiences. *Annual Review of Organizational Psychology and Organizational Behavior*, *11*(1), 63–91. https://doi.org/10.1146/annurev-orgpsych-110721-045931

Ilies, R., Wagner, D., Wilson, K., Ceja, L., Johnson, M., DeRue, S., & Ilgen, D. (2016). Flow at work and basic psychological needs: Effects on well-being. *Applied Psychology*, *66*(1), 3–24. https://doi.org/10.1111/apps.12075

Ingvarson, L., Meiers, M., & Beavis, A. (2005). Factors affecting the impact of professional development programs on teachers' knowledge, practice, student outcomes & efficacy. *Education Policy Analysis Archives*, *13*, 10. https://doi.org/10.14507/epaa.v13n10.2005

Irena, P., & Miokołaj, J. (2023). Teachers' and students' assessment of the influence of school rooms acoustic treatment on their performance and wellbeing. *Archives of Acoustics* *45*(3), 401–417. https://doi.org/10.24425/aoa.2020.134057

Itzchakov, G., Weinstein, N., Vinokur, E., & Yomtovian, A. (2022). Communicating for workplace connection: A longitudinal study of the outcomes of listening training on teachers' autonomy, psychological safety, and relational climate. *Psychology in the Schools*, *60*(4), 1279–1298. https://doi.org/10.1002/pits.22835

Jacobsson, C., Akerlund, M., Graci, E. C., & Archer, T. (2016). Team effectiveness and teachers well-being. *Clinical and Experimental Psychology*, *2*(2).

Janssen, O., & Van Yperen, N. W. (2004). Employees' goal orientations, the quality of leader-member exchange, and the outcomes of job performance and job satisfaction. *Academy of Management Journal*, *47*(3), 368–384. https://doi.org/10.2307/20159587

Jeliseh, M. T., Valizadeh, M., Zohrabi, M., & Xodabande, I. (2025). Enhancing language teachers' well-being through positive psychology interventions: A mixed-methods study focusing on gratitude journaling. *Psychology in the Schools*. https://doi.org/10.1002/pits.70005

Jellis, C., Williamson, J., & Suto, I. (2021). How well do we understand wellbeing? Teachers' experiences in an extraordinary educational era. *Research Matters*, *1*(32), 45–66. https://doi.org/10.21125/iceri.2021.1219

Jennings, P. A., Brown, J. L., Frank, J. L., Doyle, S., Oh, Y., Davis, R., Rasheed, D., DeWeese, A., DeMauro, A. A., Cham, H., & Greenberg, M. T. (2017). Impacts of the CARE for Teachers program on teachers' social and emotional competence and classroom interactions. *Journal of Educational Psychology*, *109*(7), 1010–1028. https://doi.org/10.1037/edu0000187

Jennings, P. A., Doyle, S., Oh, Y., Rasheed, D., Frank, J. L., & Brown, J. L. (2019). Long-term impacts of the CARE program on teachers' self-reported social and emotional competence and well-being. *Journal of School Psychology*, *76*, 186–202. https://doi.org/10.1016/j.jsp.2019.07.009

Jennings, P. A., & Greenberg, M. T. (2009). The prosocial classroom: Teacher social and emotional competence in relation to student and classroom outcomes. *Review of Educational Research*, *79*(1), 491–525. https://doi.org/10.3102/0034654308325693

Jepson, E., & Forrest, S. (2006). Individual contributory factors in teacher stress: The role of achievement striving and occupational commitment. *British Journal of Educational Psychology*, *76*(1), 183–197. https://doi.org/10.1348/000709905x37299

Jerrim, J., Morgan, A., & Sims, S. (2023). Teacher autonomy: Good for pupils? Good for teachers? *British Educational Research Journal*, *49*(6), 1187–1209. https://doi.org/10.1002/berj.3892

Ji, Y. (2021). Does teacher engagement matter? Exploring relationship between teachers' engagement in professional development and teaching practice. *International Journal of TESOL Studies*, *3*(4), 42–60. https://doi.org/10.46451/ijts.2021.12.04

Ji, Y. (2025). Factors affecting teachers' engagement in continuing professional development. In A. Güneyli & F. Silman (Eds.), *European proceedings of the international conference on education and educational psychology*. https://doi.org/10.15405/epiceepsy.23124.1

Jusoh, R., & Zhenni, Z. (2025). Personnel management strategies and welfare policies for enhancing teachers work–life balance and well being. *Interciencia*, *261*(3). https://doi.org/10.59671/qxjhe

Kaihoi, C. A., Bottiani, J. H., & Bradshaw, C. P. (2022). Teachers supporting teachers: A social network perspective on collegial stress support and emotional wellbeing among elementary and middle school educators. *School Mental Health*, *14*(4), 1070–1085. https://doi.org/10.1007/s12310-022-09529-y

Kamboj, K. P., & Garg, P. (2021). Teachers' psychological well-being role of emotional intelligence and resilient character traits in determining the psychological well-being of Indian school teachers. *International Journal of Educational Management*, *35*(4), 768–788. https://doi.org/10.1108/ijem-08-2019-0278

Kang, Y. T., & Printy, S. (2009). Leadership to build a democratic community within school: A case study of two Korean high schools. *Asia Pacific Education Review*, *10*(2), 237–245. https://doi.org/10.1007/s12564-009-9013-4

Karakus, M., Toprak, M., & Chen, J. (2024). Demystifying the impact of educational leadership on teachers' subjective well-being: A bibliometric analysis and literature review. *Educational Management Administration & Leadership*. https://doi.org/10.1177/17411432241242629

Karakus, M., Toprak, M., Caliskan, O., & Crawford, M. (2024). Teachers' affective and physical well-being: Emotional intelligence, emotional labour and implications for leadership. *International Journal of Educational Management*, *38*(2), 469–485. https://doi.org/10.1108/ijem-07-2023-0335

Karjalainen, S., Brännström, J. K., Christensson, J., Sahlén, B., & Lyberg-Åhlander, V. (2020). A pilot study on the relationship between primary-school teachers' well-being and the acoustics of their classrooms. *International Journal of Environmental Research and Public Health*, *17*(6), 2083. https://doi.org/10.3390/ijerph17062083

Karjalainen, S., Sahlén, B., Christensson, J., Brännström, K. J., & Lyberg Åhlander, V. (2022, January 17). Teachers' voice use and wellbeing in relation to the classroom acoustics and background noise. 10th Convention of the European Acoustics Association, Turin, Italy.

Kark, R., & Carmeli, A. (2008). Alive and creating: The mediating role of vitality and aliveness in the relationship between psychological safety and creative work involvement. *Journal of Organizational Behavior*, *30*(6), 785–804. https://doi.org/10.1002/job.571

Kasprzak, E., & Mudło-Głagolska, K. (2022). Teacher's well-being forced to work from home due to covid-19 pandemic: Work passion as a mediator. *International Journal of Environmental Research and Public Health*, *19*(22), 15095. https://doi.org/10.3390/ijerph192215095

Kelloway, E. K., Turner, N., Barling, J., & Loughlin, C. (2012). Transformational leadership and employee psychological well-being: The mediating role of employee trust in leadership. *Work & Stress*, *26*(1), 39–55. https://doi.org/10.1080/02678373.2012.660774

Kelloway, E. K., Weigand, H., McKee, M. C., & Das, H. (2012). Positive leadership and employee well-being. *Journal of Leadership & Organizational Studies*, *20*(1), 107–117. https://doi.org/10.1177/1548051812465892

Kelly, C. L., Brock, L. L., Swanson, J. D., & Russell, L. W. (2022). Teacher engagement scale for professional development. *Journal of Educational Issues*, *8*(1), 261. https://doi.org/10.5296/jei.v8i1.19636

Kennedy, Y., Flynn, N., O'Brien, E., & Greene, G. (2021). Exploring the impact of incredible years teacher classroom management training on teacher psychological outcomes. *Educational Psychology in Practice*, *37*(2), 150–168. https://doi.org/10.1080/02667363.2021.1882944

Kenzu, H. (2025, March 26). *Govt hands over houses to teachers to improve welfare*. Antara. https://tinyurl.com/4rsh5btm

Kidger, J., Brockman, R., Tilling, K., Campbell, R., Ford, T., Araya, R., King, M., & Gunnell, D. (2016). Teachers' wellbeing and depressive symptoms, and associated risk factors: A large cross sectional study in English secondary schools. *Journal of Affective Disorders*, *192*, 76–82. https://doi.org/10.1016/j.jad.2015.11.054

Kim, J., Shin, Y., Tsukayama, E., & Park, D. (2020). Stress mindset predicts job turnover among preschool teachers. *Journal of School Psychology*, *78*, 13–22. https://doi.org/10.1016/j.jsp.2019.11.002

Kim, L. E., Owusu, K., & Asbury, K. (2024). The ups and downs in perceived societal appreciation of the teaching profession during COVID-19: A longitudinal trajectory analysis. *British Educational Research Journal*, *50*(1), 93–111. https://doi.org/10.1002/berj.3914

Kim, M., & Beehr, T. A. (2017). Can empowering leaders affect subordinates' well-being and careers because they encourage subordinates' job crafting behaviors? *Journal of Leadership & Organizational Studies*, *25*(2), 184–196. https://doi.org/10.1177/1548051817727702

King, F. (2012). *Developing and sustaining teachers' professional learning: a case study of collaborative professional development* [Doctoral dissertation, University of]. https://tinyurl.com/4anfmcxd

Kingdon, G. (2010). *The impact of the sixth pay commission on teacher salaries: Assessing equity and efficiency effects*. Research Consortium on Educational Outcomes and Poverty Working Paper 20. https://tinyurl.com/375e59my

Kinman, G., Wray, S., & Strange, C. (2011). Emotional labour, burnout and job satisfaction in UK teachers: The role of workplace social support. *Educational Psychology*, *31*(7), 843–856. https://doi.org/10.1080/01443410.2011.608650

Kinnunen, U., de Bloom, J., & Virtanen, A. (2019). Do older teachers benefit more from workday break recovery than younger ones? *Scandinavian Journal of Work and Organizational Psychology*, *4*(1). https://doi.org/10.16993/sjwop.87

Klassen, R. M. (2010). Teacher stress: The mediating role of collective efficacy beliefs. *The Journal of Educational Research*, *103*(5), 342–350. https://doi.org/10.1080/00220670903383069

Klein, A. (2022, March 1). *Superficial self-care? stressed-out teachers say no thanks*. Education Week. https://tinyurl.com/2tecafnp

Kleinkorres, R., Stang-Rabrig, J., & McElvany, N. (2023). The longitudinal development of students' well-being in adolescence: The role of perceived teacher autonomy support. *Journal of Research on Adolescence*, *33*(2), 496–513. https://doi.org/10.1111/jora.12821

Klusmann, U., & Waschke, U. (2018). *Gesundheit und Wohlbefinden im Lehrberuf [Health and well-being of teachers]*. Hogrefe.

Koch, A. R., & Binnewies, C. (2015). Setting a good example: Supervisors as work–life-friendly role models within the context of boundary management. *Journal of Occupational Health Psychology*, *20*(1), 82–92. https://doi.org/10.1037/a0037890

Koon, V.-Y., & Ho, T.-S. (2021). Authentic leadership and employee engagement: The role of employee well-being. *Human Systems Management*, *40*(1), 81–92. https://doi.org/10.3233/hsm-200943

Korthagen, F. A. J., Kessels, J., Koster, B., Lagerwerf, B., & Wubbels, T. (2001). *Linking practice and theory: The pedagogy of realistic teacher education*. Lawrence Erlbaum Associates.

Kranjec, E., & Tekavc, J. (2023). The association between career anxiety and life satisfaction: The moderating role of a fixed mindset In A. Lipovec & J. Tekavc (Eds.), *Perspectives on teacher education and development* (pp. 21–37). University of Maribor, University Press. https://doi.org/10.18690/um.pef.1.2023.2

Krekel, C., Ward, G., & De Neve, J.-E. (2019). Employee wellbeing, productivity, and firm performance. *SSRN Electronic Journal*. https://doi.org/10.2139/ssrn.3356581

Kristiansen, J., Persson, R., Lund, S. P., Shibuya, H., & Nielsen, P. M. (2011). Effects of classroom acoustics and self-reported noise exposure on teachers' well-being. *Environment and Behavior*, *45*(2), 283–300. https://doi.org/10.1177/0013916511429700

Kuhn, C., Hagenauer, G., & Gröschner, A. (2022). 'Because you always learn something new yourself!' An expectancy-value-theory perspective on mentor teachers' initial motivations. *Teaching and Teacher Education*, *113*, 103659. https://doi.org/10.1016/j.tate.2022.103659

Kun, A., & Gadanecz, P. (2019). Workplace happiness, well-being and their relationship with psychological capital: A study of Hungarian Teachers. *Current Psychology*, *41*(1), 185–199. https://doi.org/10.1007/s12144-019-00550-0

Kunter, M., Klusmann, U., Baumert, J., Richter, D., Voss, T., & Hachfeld, A. (2013). Professional competence of teachers: Effects on instructional quality and student development. *Journal of Educational Psychology*, *105*(3), 805–820. https://doi.org/10.1037/a0032583

Kwatubana, S., & Molaodi, V. (2021). *Leadership styles that would enable school leaders to support the well being of teachers during COVID-19* [Paper presentation]. Bulgarian Comparative Education Society, Sofia, Bulgaria. https://t1p.de/61a6t

Labarthe-Carrara, J., Salanova, M., & Llorens, S. (2024). Trust as a driver of teacher well-being during the COVID-19 pandemic. *Revista Latinoamericana de Psicología*, *56*, 92–100. https://doi.org/10.14349/rlp.2024.v56.10

Lauth-Lebens, M., & Lauth, G. W. (2016). Behavioural modification and classroom management skills as protective factors against mental health problems in teachers: A synthesis of research. *Journal of Mental Disorders and Treatment*, 2(1). https://t1p.de/6azsv

Lawrence, D. F., Loi, N. M., & Gudex, B. W. (2018). Understanding the relationship between work intensification and burnout in secondary teachers. *Teachers and Teaching*, *25*(2), 189–199. https://doi.org/10.1080/13540602.2018.1544551

Lazarides, R., & Schiepe-Tiska, A. (2022). Heterogenität motivationaler Merkmale im Unterrichtskontext [Heterogeneity of motivational characteristics in the classroom context]. *Zeitschrift für Erziehungswissenschaft*, *25*(2), 249–267. https://doi.org/10.1007/s11618-022-01082-3

Lazarus, R., & Folkman, S. (1984). *Stress, appraisal, and coping*. Springer.

Leckey, Y., Hyland, L., Hickey, G., Lodge, A., Kelly, P., Bywater, T., Comiskey, C., Donnelly, M., & McGilloway, S. (2016). A mixed-methods evaluation of the longer-term implementation and utility of a teacher classroom management training programme in Irish primary schools. *Irish Educational Studies*, *35*(1), 35–55. https://doi.org/10.1080/03323315.2016.1147974

Lee, E. O., Lacey, H. M., Van Valkenburg, S., McGinnis, E., Huber, B. J., Benner, G. J., & Strycker, L. A. (2023). What about me? The importance of teacher social and emotional learning and well-being in the classroom. *Beyond Behavior*, *32*(1), 53–62. https://doi.org/10.1177/10742956221145942

Lee, M. H., & Swaner, L. E. (2023). Supportive leadership, teacher wellness, and school promotion. *Journal of Research on Christian Education*, *32*(3), 131–140. https://doi.org/10.1080/10656219.2023.2284798

Lei, Y. (2024). The interplay of job embeddedness, collective efficacy, and work meaningfulness on teacher well-being: A mixed-methods study with digital ethnography in China. *Frontiers in Psychology*, *15*. https://doi.org/10.3389/fpsyg.2024.1448446

Lestari, I., Sukmalana, S., Suherman, A. R., & Titi, T. (2023). The influence of achievement motivation and work discipline on employee performance. *Majalah Bisnis & IPTEK*, *16*(1), 172–180. https://doi.org/10.55208/bistek

Li, P.-H., Mayer, D., & Malmberg, L.-E. (2022). Teacher well-being in the classroom: A micro-longitudinal study. *Teaching and Teacher Education*, *115*, 103720. https://doi.org/10.1016/j.tate.2022.103720

Liang, W., Song, H., & Sun, R. (2020). Can a professional learning community facilitate teacher well-being in China? The mediating role of teaching self-efficacy. *Educational Studies*, *48*, 1–20. https://doi.org/10.1080/03055698.2020.1755953

Lima, L., de Oliveira Martins, A., Estrela, E., & Duarte, R. S. (2024). Challenges posed to leadership: Systematic review based on the relationships between curricular autonomy and teachers' well-being. *Frontiers in Education*, *9*. https://doi.org/10.3389/feduc.2024.1520947

Lindqvist, P., & Nordänger, U. K. (2006). Who dares to disconnect in the age of uncertainty? Teachers' recesses and 'off-the-clock' work. *Teachers and Teaching*, *12*(6), 623–637. https://doi.org/10.1080/13540600601029637

Liu, J. (2020). Exploring teacher attrition in urban China through interplay of wages and well-being. *Education and Urban Society*, *53*(7), 807–830. https://doi.org/10.1177/0013124520958410

Liu, L., Fathi, J., Allahveysi, S. P., & Kamran, K. (2023). A model of teachers' growth mindset, teaching enjoyment, work engagement, and teacher grit among EFL teachers. *Frontiers in Psychology*, *14*. https://doi.org/10.3389/fpsyg.2023.1137357

Liu, Y., & Keller, R. T. (2021). How psychological safety impacts & project teams' performance. *Research-Technology Management*, *64*(2), 39–45. https://doi.org/10.1080/08956308.2021.1863111

Liu, J., Siu, O. L., & Shi, K. (2010). Transformational leadership and employee well-being: The mediating role of trust in the leader and self-efficacy. *Applied Psychology*, *59*(3), 454–479. https://doi.org/10.1111/j.1464-0597.2009.00407.x

Lowery, K. (2019). Educators' perceptions of the value of coach mindset development for their well-being. *International Journal of Mentoring and Coaching in Education*, *8*(4), 310–324. https://doi.org/10.1108/ijmce-02-2019-0032

Lutz, S., Schneider, F. M., & Vorderer, P. (2020). On the downside of mobile communication: An experimental study about the influence of setting-inconsistent pressure on employees' emotional well-being. *Computers in Human Behavior*, *105*, 106216. https://doi.org/10.1016/j.chb.2019.106216

Lyubykh, Z., Gulseren, D., Premji, Z., Wingate, T. G., Deng, C., Bélanger, L. J., & Turner, N. (2022). Role of work breaks in well-being and performance: A systematic review and future research agenda. *Journal of Occupational Health Psychology*, *27*(5), 470–487. https://doi.org/10.1037/ocp0000337

Magyar-Moe, J. L. (2014). Applications of positive psychology to individual therapy. In A. C. Parks & S. M. Schueller (Eds.), *The Wiley Blackwell handbook of positive psychological interventions* (pp. 255–272). Wiley Blackwell. https://doi.org/10.1002/9781118315927.ch14

Mahenthiran Aloysius, S. M., & Christy, S. M. (2012). Self motivation for achievement and its impact on the employees' performance and satisfaction. *SSRN Electronic Journal*. https://doi.org/10.2139/ssrn.2186389

Mairitsch, A., Babic, S., Mercer, S., Sulis, G., & Shin, S. (2023). The role of compassion during the shift to online teaching for language teacher wellbeing. *Theory and Practice of Second Language Acquisition*, *9*(1), 1–22. https://doi.org/10.31261/tapsla.13123

Makki, A., & Abid, M. (2017). Influence of intrinsic and extrinsic motivation on employee's task performance. *Studies in Asian Social Science*, *4*(1), 38. https://doi.org/10.5430/sass.v4n1p38

Malinowski, P., & Lim, H. J. (2015). Mindfulness at work: Positive affect, hope, and optimism mediate the relationship between dispositional mindfulness, work engagement, and well-being. *Mindfulness*, *6*(6), 1250–1262. https://doi.org/10.1007/s12671-015-0388-5

Manda, F. (2021, February 23). *How I changed from a fixed to a growth mindset*. Commonwealth Education Trust. https://tinyurl.com/5ytpzwbu

Manning, A., Brock, R., & Emma, T. (2020). Responding to research: An interview study of the teacher wellbeing support being offered in ten English schools. *Journal of Social Science Education*, *19*(2). https://doi.org/10.4119/jsse-3312

Marcionetti, J., & Castelli, L. (2022). The job and life satisfaction of teachers: A social cognitive model integrating teachers' burnout, self-efficacy, dispositional optimism, and social support. *International Journal for Educational and Vocational Guidance*, *23*(2), 441–463. https://doi.org/10.1007/s10775-021-09516-w

Margolis, J., Hodge, A., & Alexandrou, A. (2014). The teacher educator's role in promoting institutional versus individual teacher well-being. *Journal of Education for Teaching*, *40*(4), 391–408. https://doi.org/10.1080/02607476.2014.929382

Maricuţoiu, L. P., Pap, Z., Ştefancu, E., Mladenovici, V., Valache, D. G., Popescu, B. D., Ilie, M., & Vîrgă, D. (2023). Is teachers' well-being associated with students' school experience? A meta-analysis of cross-sectional evidence. *Educational Psychology Review*, *35*(1), 1–36. https://doi.org/10.1007/s10648-023-09721-9

Marlow, R., Hansford, L., Edwards, V., Ukoumunne, O. C., Norman, S., Ingarfield, S., Sharkey, S., Logan, S., & Ford, T. (2015). Teaching classroom management: A potential public health intervention? *Health Education*, *115*(3/4), 230–248. https://doi.org/10.1108/he-03-2014-0030

Mat Zin, N. I., Zainudin, Z. N., & Sulong, R. M. (2023). Relationship between resilience and school culture with psychological well-being of school teachers. *International Journal of Academic Research in Business and Social Sciences*, *13*(12). https://doi.org/10.6007/ijarbss/v13-i12/20381

Matos, M., Albuquerque, I., Galhardo, A., Cunha, M., Pedroso Lima, M., Palmeira, L., Petrocchi, N., McEwan, K., Maratos, F. A., & Gilbert, P. (2022). Nurturing compassion in schools: A randomized controlled trial of the effectiveness of a Compassionate Mind Training program for teachers. *PLoS One*, *17*(3), e0263480. https://doi.org/10.1371/journal.pone.0263480

Mavi, D., Tuti, G., & Ozdemir, M. (2024). How does teacher academic optimism affect teacher self-efficacy: Mediating role of teacher professional development and teacher subjective well-being? *Psychology in the Schools*, *62*(4), 1013–1025. https://doi.org/10.1002/pits.23373

McCallum, F. (2020). The changing nature of teachers' work and its impact on wellbeing. In M. A. White & F. McCallum (Eds.), *Critical perspectives on teaching, learning and leadership: Enhancing educational outcomes* (pp. 17–44). Springer Singapore. https://doi.org/10.1007/978-981-15-6667-7_2

McLean, L., Abry, T., Taylor, M., & Gaias, L. (2020). The influence of adverse classroom and school experiences on first year teachers' mental health and career optimism. *Teaching and Teacher Education*, *87*, 102956. https://doi.org/10.1016/j.tate.2019.102956

McQuade, L. (2024). Factors affecting secondary teacher wellbeing in England: Self-perceptions, policy and politics. *British Educational Research Journal*, *50*(3), 1367–1395. https://doi.org/10.1002/berj.3973

Mealings, K., Maggs, L., & Buchholz, J. M. (2024). The effects of classroom acoustic conditions on teachers' health and well-being: A scoping review. *Journal of Speech, Language, and Hearing Research*, *67*(1), 346–367. https://doi.org/10.1044/2023_jslhr-23-00256

Meidelina, O., Saleh, A. Y., Cathlin, C. A., & Winesa, S. A. (2023). Transformational leadership and teacher well-being: A systematic review. *Journal of Education and Learning (EduLearn)*, *17*(3), 417–424. https://doi.org/10.11591/edulearn.v17i3.20858

Mennes, H., von der Embse, N., Kim, E., Sundar, P., Hines, D., & Welliver, M. (2024). Are 'well' teachers 'better' teachers? A look into the relationship between first-year teacher emotion and use of evidence-based instructional strategies. *School Psychology*, *39*(3), 325–335. https://doi.org/10.1037/spq0000593

Mikus, K., & Teoh, K. R. H. (2021). Psychological capital, future-oriented coping, and the well-being of secondary school teachers in Germany. *Educational Psychology*, *42*(3), 334–353. https://doi.org/10.1080/01443410.2021.1954601

Milatz, A., Lüftenegger, M., & Schober, B. (2015). Teachers' relationship closeness with students as a resource for teacher wellbeing: A response surface analytical approach. *Frontiers in Psychology*, *6*. https://doi.org/10.3389/fpsyg.2015.01949

Min, A. W. (2024, September 23). *'Very challenging' to deal with parents who expect immediate responses to messages: Teachers*. CNA. https://tinyurl.com/wkwb9be9

Ministry of Education Singapore. (2022). *MOE strengthens teacher well-being initiatives*. https://www.moe.gov.sg/news/press-releases/moe-strengthens-teacher-well-being-initiatives

Moè, A., & Katz, I. (2020). Self-compassionate teachers are more autonomy supportive and structuring whereas self-derogating teachers are more controlling and chaotic: The mediating role of need satisfaction and burnout. *Teaching and Teacher Education*, *96*, 103173. https://doi.org/10.1016/j.tate.2020.103173

Moè, A., Pazzaglia, F., & Ronconi, L. (2010). When being able is not enough. The combined value of positive affect and self-efficacy for job satisfaction in teaching. *Teaching and Teacher Education*, *26*, 1145–1153. https://doi.org/10.1016/j.tate.2010.02.010

Moeller, C., & Chung-Yan, G. A. (2013). Effects of social support on professors' work stress. *International Journal of Educational Management*, *27*(3), 188–202. https://doi.org/10.1108/09513541311306431

Moen, P., Kelly, E. L., Fan, W., Lee, S.-R., Almeida, D., Kossek, E. E., & Buxton, O. M. (2016). Does a flexibility/support organizational initiative improve high-tech employees' well-being? Evidence from the work, family, and health network. *American Sociological Review*, *81*(1), 134–164. https://doi.org/10.1177/0003122415622391

Molyneux, T. M. (2021). Preparing teachers for emotional labour: The missing piece in teacher education. *Journal of Teaching and Learning*, *15*(1), 39–56. https://doi.org/10.22329/jtl.v15i1.6333

Morgan, M., Kitching, K., & O'Leary, M. (2007). *The psychic rewards of teaching: Examining global, national and local influences on teacher motivation* [Paper presentation]. AERA Annual Meeting, Chicago.

Morris, I. (2015). *Teaching happiness and well-being in schools: Learning to ride elephants*. Bloomsbury Publishing.

Mouza, C. (2009). Does research-based professional development make a difference? A longitudinal investigation of teacher learning in technology integration. *Teachers College Record: The Voice of Scholarship in Education*, *111*(5), 1195–1241. https://doi.org/10.1177/016146810911100502

MTI-Hungary Today. (2023, May 11). *Teachers set to receive salary increase from January 2024*. Hungary Today. https://hungarytoday.hu/government-plans-to-increase-teacher-salaries-20-21-by-2025/?utm_source=chatgpt.com

Murturi, D. (2024). The relationship between teachers' emotional intelligence on job burnout and teaching effectiveness. *International Journal of Management Studies and Social Science Research*, *06*(04), 304–311. https://doi.org/10.56293/ijmsssr.2024.5130

Mushtaq, A., & Mehmood, H. (2023). Impact of job crafting intervention on psychological empowerment, work engagement, and affective well-being in teachers. *Journal of Professional & Applied Psychology*, *4*(2), 98–116. https://doi.org/10.52053/jpap.v4i2.138

Naghieh, Ali, Bonell, P., Thompson, C. P., Aber, M., & Lawrence, J. (2015). Organisational interventions for improving wellbeing and reducing work-related stress in teachers *Cochrane Database of Systematic Reviews*. Wiley.

Nagy, E., Takács, I., & Czabán, C. (2024). Being well and striving steady at work: The relationship of social support and self-concordant goal selection with teacher burnout. *Acta Polytechnica Hungarica*, *21*(3), 9–24. https://doi.org/10.12700/aph.21.3.2024.3.2

Nalipay, M., King, R., Mordeno, I., & Wang, H. (2021). Are good teachers born or made? Teachers who hold a growth mindset about their teaching ability have better well-being. *Educational Psychology*, *42*, 1–19. https://doi.org/10.1080/01443410.2021.2001791

Nalipay, M., Mordeno, I., Semilla, J. r., & Frondozo, C. (2019). Implicit beliefs about teaching ability, teacher emotions, and teaching satisfaction. *The Asia-Pacific Education Researcher*, *28*. https://doi.org/10.1007/s40299-019-00467-z

Näring, G., Briët, M., & Brouwers, A. (2006). Beyond demand–control: Emotional labour and symptoms of burnout in teachers. *Work & Stress*, *20*(4), 303–315. https://doi.org/10.1080/02678370601065182

National Institute of Education. (2021). *A school-wide approach to well-being*. SingTeach. https://singteach.nie.edu.sg/2022/01/10/st79-a-school-wide-approach-to-well-being/

Nazari, M., & Karimpour, S. (2024). Exploring Iranian EAP teachers' well-being: An activity theory perspective. *Asian-Pacific Journal of Second and Foreign Language Education*, *9*(1). https://doi.org/10.1186/s40862-023-00249-7

New Zealand Council for Educational Research. (2018). *Educational leadership capability framework*. https://tinyurl.com/4rsmudtk

Nicolosi, S., Alba, M., & Pitrolo, C. (2023). Primary school teachers' emotions, implicit beliefs, and self-efficacy during the COVID-19 pandemic. *Frontiers in Sports and Active Living*, *4*. https://doi.org/10.3389/fspor.2022.1064072

Nicuță, E. G., Diaconu-Gherasim, L. R., & Constantin, T. (2022). How trait gratitude relates to teachers' burnout and work engagement: Job demands and resources as mediators. *Current Psychology*, *42*(34), 30338–30347. https://doi.org/10.1007/s12144-022-04086-8

Nie, Y., Chua, B. L., Yeung, A. S., Ryan, R. M., & Chan, W. Y. (2014). The importance of autonomy support and the mediating role of work motivation for well-being: Testing self-determination theory in a Chinese work organisation. *International Journal of Psychology*, *50*(4), 245–255. https://doi.org/10.1002/ijop.12110

Nordgren, K., Kristiansson, M., Liljekvist, Y., & Bergh, D. (2021). Collegial collaboration when planning and preparing lessons: A large-scale study exploring the conditions and infrastructure for teachers' professional development. *Teaching and Teacher Education*, *108*, 103513. https://doi.org/10.1016/j.tate.2021.103513

Norlander, T., Moås, L., & Archer, T. (2005). Noise and stress in primary and secondary school children: Noise reduction and increased concentration ability through a short but regular exercise and relaxation program. *School Effectiveness and School Improvement*, *16*(1), 91–99. https://doi.org/10.1080/09243450500114173

Nwoko, J. C., Emeto, T. I., Malau-Aduli, A. E. O., & Malau-Aduli, B. S. (2023). A systematic review of the factors that influence teachers' occupational wellbeing. *International Journal of Environmental Research and Public Health*, *20*(12), 6070. https://doi.org/10.3390/ijerph20126070

O'Hara-Gregan, J. (2023). Supporting early childhood teacher well-being through the practice of mindful self-compassion. *Australasian Journal of Early Childhood*, *48*(4), 319–331. https://doi.org/10.1177/18369391231202833

O'Neill, A., Baldwin, D., Cortese, S., & Sinclair, J. (2022). Impact of intrawork rest breaks on doctors' performance and well-being: systematic review. *BMJ Open*, *12*(12), e062469. https://doi.org/10.1136/bmjopen-2022-062469

O'Reilly, P. E. (2014). *Teachers at work: Factors influencing satisfaction, retention and the professional well-being of elementary and secondary educators* [Doctoral dissertation, City of New York University]. CUNY Academic Works. https://academicworks.cuny.edu/gc_etds/88

Oh, J. H., Tygret, J. A., & Mendez, S. L. (2024). The benefits of being a mentor teacher in a teacher residency program. *International Journal of Mentoring and Coaching in Education*, *13*(2), 214–229. https://doi.org/10.1108/ijmce-06-2023-0048

Olčar, D., Rijavec, M., & Ljubin Golub, T. (2019). Primary school teachers' life satisfaction: The role of life goals, basic psychological needs and flow at work. *Current Psychology*, *38*(2), 320–329. https://doi.org/10.1007/s12144-017-9611-y

Ololube, N. (2006). Teachers job satisfaction and motivation for school effectiveness: An assessment. *Essays in Education*, *18*(1), 1–19.

Önder, Ş. (2019). Analyzing effect of teachers personal empowerment perceptions to their passion for working by various factors. *Educational Research and Reviews*, *14*(12), 419–433. https://doi.org/10.5897/err2017.3173

Organisation for Economic Co-operation and Development (OECD). (2019). *OECD future of education and skills 2030: OECD Learning Compass 2030*. https://www.oecd.org/en/about/projects/future-of-education-and-skills-2030.html

Organisation for Economic Co-operation and Development (OECD). (2022). *Review of inclusive education in Portugal, Reviews of national policies for education*. OECD Publishing. https://doi.org/10.1787/a9c95902-en

Orland-Barak, L. (2001). Learning to mentor as learning a second language of teaching. *Cambridge Journal of Education*, *31*(1), 53–68. https://doi.org/10.1080/03057640123464

Ortan, F., Simut, C., & Simut, R. (2021). Self-efficacy, job satisfaction and teacher well-being in the K–12 educational system. *International Journal of Environmental Research and Public Health*, *18*(23), 12763. https://doi.org/10.3390/ijerph182312763

Ostermeier, T. C. J., Koops, W., & Peccei, R. (2023). Effects of job demands and resources on the subjective well-being of teachers. *Review of Education*, *11*(3). https://doi.org/10.1002/rev3.3416

Ouweneel, E., Le Blanc, P. M., & Schaufeli, W. B. (2013). Do-it-yourself. *Career Development International*, *18*(2), 173–195. https://doi.org/10.1108/cdi-10-2012-0102

Page, K. (2005). *Subjective wellbeing in the workplace* [Bachelor-Thesis, Deakin University]. https://t1p.de/xtwfm

Page, K. M., & Vella-Brodrick, D. A. (2012). The working for wellness program: RCT of an employee well-being intervention. *Journal of Happiness Studies*, *14*(3), 1007–1031. https://doi.org/10.1007/s10902-012-9366-y

Paletta, A. (2014). Improving students' learning through school autonomy: Evidence from the international civic and citizenship survey. *Journal of School Choice*, *8*(3), 381–409. https://doi.org/10.1080/15582159.2014.942173

Pan, H.-L. W., Chung, C.-H., & Lin, Y.-C. (2023). Exploring the predictors of teacher well-being: An analysis of teacher training preparedness, autonomy, and workload. *Sustainability*, *15*(7), 5804. https://doi.org/10.3390/su15075804

Pearson, L., & Moomaw, W. (2005). The relationship between teacher autonomy and stress, work satisfaction, empowerment, and professionalism. *Educational Research Quarterly*, *29*(1), 38–54.

Pedro, N., Baeta, P., Paio, A., Pedro, A., & Matos, J. F. (2017). *Redesigning classrooms for the future: Gathering inputs from students, teachers and designers.* 11th International Technology, Education and Development Conference.

Peláez-Fernández, M. A., Mérida-López, S., Sánchez-Álvarez, N., & Extremera, N. (2021). Managing teachers' job attitudes: The potential benefits of being a happy and emotional intelligent teacher. *Frontiers in Psychology*, *12*. https://doi.org/10.3389/fpsyg.2021.661151

Peng, W., Liu, Y., & Peng, J.-E. (2023). Feeling and acting in classroom teaching: The relationships between teachers' emotional labor, commitment, and well-being. *System*, *116*, 103093. https://doi.org/10.1016/j.system.2023.103093

Perry, N. E., Brenner, C., Collie, R. J., & Hofer, G. (2015). Thriving on challenge: Examining one teacher's view on sources of support for motivation and well-being. *Exceptionality Education International*, *25*(1). https://doi.org/10.5206/eei.v25i1.7715

Persson, M., & Thunman, E. (2017). Boundary practices and social media: The case of teachers' use of Facebook to communicate with pupils. *HUMAN IT*, *13*(3), 24–48.

Pfister, I. B. (2019). *Appreciation at work and its consequences* [Doctoral Thesis, Universität Bern]. BORIS Theses. https://boristheses.unibe.ch/id/eprint/1367

Pfister, I. B., Jacobshagen, N., Kälin, W., & Semmer, N. K. (2020). How does appreciation lead to higher job satisfaction? *Journal of Managerial Psychology*, *35*(6), 465–479. https://doi.org/10.1108/JMP-12-2018-0555

Philipp, A., & Schüpbach, H. (2010). Longitudinal effects of emotional labour on emotional exhaustion and dedication of teachers. *Journal of Occupational Health Psychology*, *15*(4), 494–504. https://doi.org/10.1037/a0021046

Pluut, H., & Wonders, J. (2020). Not able to lead a healthy life when you need it the most: Dual role of lifestyle behaviors in the association of blurred work–life boundaries with well-being. *Frontiers in Psychology*, *11*. https://doi.org/10.3389/fpsyg.2020.607294

Pohling, R., & Diessner, R. (2016). Moral elevation and moral beauty: A review of the empirical literature. *Review of General Psychology*, *20*(4), 412–425. https://doi.org/10.1037/gpr0000089

Poortvliet, P. M., Anseel, F., & Theuwis, F. (2015). Mastery-approach and mastery-avoidance goals and their relation with exhaustion and engagement at work: The roles of emotional and instrumental support. *Work & Stress*, *29*(2), 150–170. https://doi.org/10.1080/02678373.2015.1031856

Poulou, M. S. (2020). Students' adjustment at school: The role of teachers' need satisfaction, teacher–student relationships and student well-being. *School Psychology International*, *41*(6), 499–521. https://doi.org/10.1177/0143034320951911

Price, D., & McCallum, F. (2015). Ecological influences on teachers' well-being and 'fitness'. *Asia-Pacific Journal of Teacher Education*, *43*(3), 195–209. https://doi.org/10.1080/1359866X.2014.932329

Price, W., & Terry, E. (2008). Can small class sizes help retain teachers to the profession? *International Journal of Educational Leadership Preparation*, *3*(2), 1–5.

Prout, P., Lowe, G., Gray, C., & Jefferson, S. (2019). An elixir for veteran teachers: The power of social connections in keeping these teachers passionate and enthusiastic in their work. *The Qualitative Report*, *24*(9), 2244–2258. https://doi.org/10.46743/2160-3715/2019.4038

Rafsanjani, M. A., Pamungkas, H. P., & Rahmawati, E. D. (2019). Does teacher–student relationship mediate the relation between student misbehavior and teacher psychological well-being? *Journal of Accounting and Business Education*, *4*(1), 34. https://doi.org/10.26675/jabe.v4i1.8411

Rahm, T., & Heise, E. (2019). Teaching happiness to teachers: Development and evaluation of a training in subjective well-being. *Frontiers in Psychology*, *10*(27/03). https://doi.org/10.3389/fpsyg.2019.02703

Rajabi, M., & Ghezelsefloo, M. (2020). The relationship between job stress and job-related affective well-being among English language teachers: The moderating role of self- compassion. *Iranian Journal of English for Academic Purposes*, *9*(1), 95–105.

Ransford, C. R., Greenberg, M., Domitrovich, C., Small, M. L., & Jacobson, L. (2009). The role of teachers' psychological experiences and perceptions of curriculum supports on the implementation of a social and emotional learning curriculum. *School Psychology Review*, *38*(4), 510–532.

Rasheed-Karim, W. (2020). The Influence of policy on emotional labour and burnout among further and adult education teachers in the UK. *International Journal of Emerging Technologies in Learning*, *15*(24), 232. https://doi.org/10.3991/ijet.v15i24.19307

Rawling, C. (2016, November 1). *The selfish teacher*. ImaginED. https://tinyurl.com/f9dfe7m5

Ray, E. B., & Miller, K. I. (1991). The influence of communication structure and social support on job stress and burnout. *Management Communication Quarterly*, *4*(4), 506–527. https://doi.org/10.1177/0893318991004004005

Raza, M. Y., Akhtar, M. W., Husnain, M., & Akhtar, M. S. (2015). The impact of intrinsic motivation on employee's job satisfaction. *Management and Organizational Studies*, *2*(3), 80–88. https://doi.org/10.5430/mos.v2n3p80

Reinke, K., & Gerlach, G. I. (2021). Linking availability expectations, bidirectional boundary management behavior and preferences, and employee well-being: An integrative study approach. *Journal of Business and Psychology*, *37*(4), 695–715. https://doi.org/10.1007/s10869-021-09768-x

Rexroth, M., Michel, A., & Bosch, C. (2017). Promoting well-being by teaching employees how to segment their life domains. *Zeitschrift für*

Arbeits- und Organisationspsychologie A&O, *61*(4), 197–212. https://doi.org/10.1026/0932-4089/a000253

Richter, E., Lazarides, R., & Richter, D. (2021). Four reasons for becoming a teacher educator: A large-scale study on teacher educators' motives and well-being. *Teaching and Teacher Education*, *102*, 103322. https://doi.org/10.1016/j.tate.2021.103322

Right to Play. (2025). *Changing the game: Dela's story*. https://tinyurl.com/6f74r4fv

Rinas, R., Dresel, M., & Daumiller, M. (2020). Faculty subjective well-being: An achievement goal approach. *Educational Research*, *115*, 1–15. https://doi.org/10.31234/osf.io/gqyuj

Rinas, R., Kiltz, L., Dresel, M., & Daumiller, M. (2023). How university instructors' achievement goals are related to subjective well-being: A cross-lagged panel analysis. *Journal of Educational Psychology*, *115*(8), 1141–1157. https://doi.org/10.1037/edu0000809

Rivkin, W., Diestel, S., & Schmidt, K.-H. (2018). Which daily experiences can foster well-being at work? A diary study on the interplay between flow experiences, affective commitment, and self-control demands. *Journal of Occupational Health Psychology*, *23*(1), 99–111. https://doi.org/10.1037/ocp0000039

Robinette, R. L. (2024). Recognizing teacher well-being as essential for professional development. *Current Issues in Education*, *25*(2). https://doi.org/10.14507/cie.vol25iss2.2204

Roeder, P. M. (1991). Der Lehrer als Einzelkämpfer. Lehrerindividualismus und Schulkultur [The teacher as a lone fighter: Teacher individualism and school culture]. In S. Bäuerle (Ed.), *Lehrer auf der Schulbank. Vorschläge für eine zeitgemäße Lehreraus- und -fortbildung. [Teachers on the school bench: Proposals for contemporary teacher education and professional development]* (pp. 77–87). Metzler.

Roeser, R. W., Schonert-Reichl, K. A., Jha, A., Cullen, M., Wallace, L., Wilensky, R., Oberle, E., Thomson, K., Taylor, C., & Harrison, J. (2013). Mindfulness training and reductions in teacher stress and burnout: Results from two randomized, waitlist-control field trials. *Journal of Educational Psychology*, *105*(3), 787–804. https://doi.org/10.1037/a0032093

Roeser, R. W., Skinner, E., Beers, J., & Jennings, P. A. (2012). Mindfulness training and teachers' professional development: An emerging area of research and practice. *Child Development Perspectives*, 6(2), 167–173. https://doi.org/10.1111/j.1750-8606.2012.00238.x

Roethlisberger, F. J., & Dickson, W. J. (1939). *Management and the worker*. Harvard University Press.

Roffey, S. (2012). Pupil wellbeing–teacher wellbeing: Two sides of the same coin? *Educational and Child Psychology*, *29*(4), 8–17. https://doi.org/10.53841/bpsecp.2012.29.4.8

Rosales, R. M. (2016). Energizing social interactions at work: An exploration of relationships that generate employee and organizational thriving. *Open Journal of Social Sciences*, *04*(09), 29–33. https://doi.org/10.4236/jss.2016.49004

Ross, S. W., Romer, N., & Horner, R. H. (2011). Teacher well-being and the implementation of school-wide positive behavior interventions and supports. *Journal of Positive Behavior Interventions*, *14*(2), 118–128. https://doi.org/10.1177/1098300711413820

Rundle-Gardiner, A. C., & Carr, S. (2005). Quitting a workplace that discourages achievement motivation: Do Individual differences matter? *New Zealand Journal of Psychology*, *34*, 149–156.

Russell, D. W., Altmaier, E., & Van Velzen, D. (1987). Job-related stress, social support, and burnout among classroom teachers. *Journal of Applied Psychology*, 72(2), 269–274. https://doi.org/10.1037/0021-9010.72.2.269

Ryff, C. D. (1989). Happiness is everything, or is it? Explorations on the meaning of psychological well-being. *Journal of Personality and Social Psychology*, *57*(6), 1069–1081. https://doi.org/10.1037/0022-3514.57.6.1069

Saleem, J. (2024, n.d.). *Rethinking teacher wellbeing: Beyond stress and burnout*. Azim Premji University. https://azimpremjiuniversity.edu.in/rethinking-teacher-wellbeing-beyond-stress-and-burnout

Saleh, A. Y., Kurniawati, F., Salim, R. M. A., & Poerwandari, E. K. (2015). Factors influencing the well-being of primary school teachers in Indonesia: A pilot study. *Psychological Research on Urban Society*, 7(1), 12–24. https://doi.org/10.7454/proust.v7i1.1140

Santos, A., Hayward, T., & Ramos, H. M. (2012). Organizational culture, work and personal goals as predictors of employee well-being. *Journal of Organizational Culture, Communications and Conflict*, *16*, 1–25.

Sarros, J. C., & Sarros, A. M. (1992). Social support and teacher burnout. *Journal of Educational Administration*, *30*(1). https://doi.org/10.1108/09578239210008826

Schiefele, U., Streblow, L., & Retelsdorf, J. (2013). Dimensions of teacher interest and their relations to occupational well-being and instructional practices. *Journal for Educational Research Online*, *5*(1), 7–37. https://doi.org/10.25656/01:8018

Schnall, S., Roper, J., & Fessler, D. M. (2010). Elevation leads to altruistic behavior. *Psychological Science*, *21*(3), 315–320. https://doi.org/10.1177/0956797609359882

Schön Persson, S., Nilsson Lindström, P., Pettersson, P., Nilsson, M., & Blomqvist, K. (2018). Resources for work-related well-being: A qualitative study about healthcare employees' experiences of relationships at work. *Journal of Clinical Nursing*, *27*(23–24), 4302–4310. https://doi.org/10.1111/jocn.14543

Schonfeld, I. (2001). Stress in 1st-year women teachers: The context of social support and coping. *Genetic Social and General Psychology Monographs*, *127*(2), 133–168.

Schulte, P., & Vainio, H. (2010). Well-being at work: Overview and perspective. *Scandinavian Journal of Work, Environment & Health*, *36*(5), 422–429. http://www.jstor.org/stable/40967878

Seiza, J., Vossb, T., & Kuntera, M. (2015). When knowing is not enough: The relevance of teachers' cognitive and emotional resources for classroom management. *Frontline Learning Research*, *3*(1), 55–77.

Seligman, M. E. P. (2011). *Flourish: A visionary new understanding of happiness and well-being*. Free Press.

Senarathna, W. A. N. M., & Ranasinghe, V. R. (2024). The influence of emotional work on employee well-being: Mediating effect of perceived organizational support. *Journal of Business Studies*, *11*(2), 37–56. https://doi.org/10.4038/jbs.v11i2.107

Shen, B., McCaughtry, N., Martin, J., Garn, A., Kulik, N., & Fahlman, M. (2015). The relationship between teacher burnout and student motivation. *British Journal of Educational Psychology*, *85*(4), 519–532. https://doi.org/10.1111/bjep.12089

Shim, S. S., Cho, Y., & Cassady, J. (2013). Goal structures: The role of teachers' achievement goals and theories of intelligence. *The Journal of*

Experimental Education, *81*(1), 84–104. https://doi.org/10.1080/00220973.2011.635168

Shoshani, A. (2021). Growth mindset in the maths classroom: A key to teachers' well-being and effectiveness. *Teachers and Teaching*, 27, 1–23. https://doi.org/10.1080/13540602.2021.2007370

Shoukat, A. (2024). Impact of physical infrastructure and learning resources on teacher quality. *Kashf Journal of Multidisciplinary Research*, *1*(10), 40–48. https://doi.org/10.71146/kjmr109

Sianoja, M., Syrek, C. J., de Bloom, J., Korpela, K., & Kinnunen, U. (2018). Enhancing daily well-being at work through lunchtime park walks and relaxation exercises: Recovery experiences as mediators. *Journal of Occupational Health Psychology*, *23*(3), 428–442. https://doi.org/10.1037/ocp0000083

Siemsen, E., Roth, A. V., Balasubramanian, S., & Anand, G. (2009). The influence of psychological safety and confidence in knowledge on employee knowledge sharing. *Manufacturing & Service Operations Management*, *11*(3), 429–447. https://doi.org/10.1287/msom.1080.0233

Singh, B., Winkel, D. E., & Selvarajan, T. T. (2013). Managing diversity at work: Does psychological safety hold the key to racial differences in employee performance? *Journal of Occupational and Organizational Psychology*, *86*(2), 242–263. https://doi.org/10.1111/joop.12015

Singh, P. (2024). *Pooja Singh: Patna CBCT Training*. Global Compassion Coalition. https://www.globalcompassioncoalition.org/compassion-corp/pooja-singh/

Skaalvik, E. M., & Skaalvik, S. (2011). Teachers' feeling of belonging, exhaustion, and job satisfaction: The role of school goal structure and value consonance. *Anxiety, Stress & Coping*, *24*(4), 369–385. https://doi.org/10.1080/10615806.2010.544300

Skaalvik, E. M., & Skaalvik, S. (2014). Teacher self-efficacy and perceived autonomy: Relations with teacher engagement, job satisfaction, and emotional exhaustion. *Psychological Reports*, *114*(1), 68–77. https://doi.org/10.2466/14.02.pr0.114k14w0

Skaalvik, E. M., & Skaalvik, S. (2019). Teacher self-efficacy and collective teacher efficacy: Relations with perceived job resources and job demands, feeling of belonging, and teacher engagement. *Creative Education*, *10*(07), 1400–1424. https://doi.org/10.4236/ce.2019.107104

Skaalvik, E. M., & Skaalvik, S. (2023). Shared goals and values in the teaching profession, job satisfaction and motivation to leave the teaching profession: The mediating role of psychological need satisfaction. *Social Psychology of Education*, *26*(5), 1227–1244. https://doi.org/10.1007/s11218-023-09787-x

Skinner, B., Leavey, G., & Rothi, D. (2019). Managerialism and teacher professional identity: Impact on well-being among teachers in the UK. *Educational Review*, *73*(1), 1–16. https://doi.org/10.1080/00131911.2018.1556205

Slemp, G. R., Vella-Brodrick, D., & Francis, J. (2023, March 9). *Research shows how 'job crafting' can help teachers manage and enjoy their stressful work*. Phys Org. https://phys.org/news/2023-03-job-crafting-teachers-enjoy-stressful.html#google_vignette

Smith, C. (2018, February 26). *Quality, not quantity: How teacher workload has been reduced by focusing on quality*. Department for Education, UK. https://tinyurl.com/evehyt9u

Smith, M. L., & Glass, G. V. (1980). Meta-analysis of research on class size and its relationship to attitudes and instruction. *American Educational Research Journal*, *17*(4), 419–433. https://doi.org/10.3102/00028312017004419

Sohail, M. M., Baghdady, A., Choi, J., Huynh, H. V., Whetten, K., & Proeschold-Bell, R. J. (2023). Factors influencing teacher wellbeing and burnout in schools: A scoping review. *Work*, *76*(4), 1317–1331. https://doi.org/10.3233/wor-220234

Soini, T., Pyhältö, K., & Pietarinen, J. (2010). Pedagogical well-being: Reflecting learning and well-being in teachers' work. *Teachers and Teaching*, *16*(6), 735–751. https://doi.org/10.1080/13540602.2010.517690

Song, H., Gu, Q., & Zhang, Z. (2020). An exploratory study of teachers' subjective wellbeing: Understanding the links between teachers' income satisfaction, altruism, self-efficacy and work satisfaction. *Teachers and Teaching*, *26*(1), 3–31. https://doi.org/10.1080/13540602.2020.1719059

Soykan, A., Gardner, D., & Edwards, T. (2019). Subjective wellbeing in New Zealand teachers: An examination of the role of psychological capital. *Journal of Psychologists and Counsellors in Schools*, *29*(2), 130–138. https://doi.org/10.1017/jgc.2019.14

Spencer, T. (2024, May 6). *Want to show teachers appreciation? This top school gives them more freedom*. AP News. https://apnews.com/article/

teacher-appreciation-week-henderson-school-florida-103044d32bde4d4a756409c34b9a2c82

Spruyt, B., Van Droogenbroeck, F., Van Den Borre, L., Emery, L., Keppens, G., & Siongers, J. (2021). Teachers' perceived societal appreciation: PISA outcomes predict whether teachers feel valued in society. *International Journal of Educational Research*, *109*, 101833. https://doi.org/10.1016/j.ijer.2021.101833

Staff Editor. (2024, June 3). *Workshop on SEE learning and cognitively based compassion training held at Dharamshala*. Administrative Training & Welfare Society. https://atws.in/school-teachers-receive-workshop-on-see-learning-and-cognitively-based-compassion-training/

Stănculescu, E. (2014). Psychological predictors and mediators of subjective well-being in a sample of Romanian teacher. *Revista de Cercetare Şi Intervenţie Socială*, *46*, 37–52.

Stark, K., Daulat, N., & King, S. P. (2022, January 24). *A vision for teachers' emotional well-being*. Kappan. https://tinyurl.com/29xkspwp

Staw, B. M., Sutton, R. I., & Pelled, L. H. (1994). Employee positive emotion and favorable outcomes at the workplace. *Organization Science*, *5*(1), 51–71. https://doi.org/10.1287/orsc.5.1.51

Stephens, J. P., Heaphy, E., & Dutton, J. E. (2012). High-quality connections. In K. S. Cameron & G. M. Spreitzer (Eds.), *The Oxford handbook of positive organizational scholarship* (pp. 385–399). Oxford University Press.

Stocker, D., Jacobshagen, N., Krings, R., Pfister, I. B., & Semmer, N. K. (2014). Appreciative leadership and employee well-being in everyday working life. *German Journal of Human Resource Management: Zeitschrift für Personalforschung*, *28*(1–2), 73–95. https://doi.org/10.1177/239700221402800105

Stocker, D., Keller, A. C., Meier, L. L., Elfering, A., Pfister, I. B., Jacobshagen, N., & Semmer, N. K. (2019). Appreciation by supervisors buffers the impact of work interruptions on well-being longitudinally. *International Journal of Stress Management*, *26*(4), 331–343. https://doi.org/10.1037/str0000111

Strahan née Brown, C., Gibbs, S., & Reid, A. (2018). The psychological environment and teachers' collective-efficacy beliefs. *Educational Psychology in Practice*, *35*(2), 147–164. https://doi.org/10.1080/02667363.2018.1547685

Taborda, R. F., Gomes, R. F., Rocha, C. H., & Samelli, A. G. (2020). Evaluation of noise reduction interventions in a school. *Folia Phoniatrica et Logopaedica*, *73*(5), 367–375. https://doi.org/10.1159/000509332

Tallinn City Government, T. (2025, February 19). *Tallinn begins reducing class sizes*. https://www.tallinn.ee/en/news/tallinn-begins-reducing-class-sizes

Tan, L. D. C., & Urdan, T. (2025). Exploring the responsibilities, boundaries, and well-being of teachers in the Philippines. *Psychology International*, *7*(1), 14. https://doi.org/10.3390/psycholint7010014

Tang, Y., He, W., Liu, L., & Li, Q. (2018). Beyond the paycheck: Chinese rural teacher well-being and the impact of professional learning and local community engagement. *Teachers and Teaching*, *24*(7), 825–839. https://doi.org/10.1080/13540602.2018.1470972

Tao, V. Y. K., Li, Y., Lam, K. H., Leung, C. W., Sun, C. I., & Wu, A. M. S. (2021). From teachers' implicit theories of intelligence to job stress: The mediating role of teachers' causal attribution of students' academic achievement. *Journal of Applied Social Psychology*, *51*(5), 522–533. https://doi.org/10.1111/jasp.12754

Tardy, C. M. (2004). 'That's why I do it': Flow and EFL teachers' practices. *ELT Journal*, *58*(2), 118–128. https://doi.org/10.1093/elt/58.2.118

Tassell, J., Gerstenschlager, N. E., Syzmanski, T., & Denning, S. (2020). A study of factors impacting elementary mathematics preservice teachers: Improving mindfulness, anxiety, self-efficacy, and mindset. *School Science and Mathematics*, *120*(6), 333–344. https://doi.org/10.1111/ssm.12425

Teacher Task Force & UNESCO. (2024). *Valuing teacher voices: Towards a new social contract for education*. https://unesdoc.unesco.org/ark:/48223/pf0000391453

Teachers Acceleration Model and Growth Coaching. (2024, April 8). *Developing a growth mindset in teachers, for continuous improvement*. So They Can. https://www.sotheycan.org/blog/teachers-growth-mindset/

Temam, S., Billaudeau, N., & Vercambre, M.-N. (2019). Burnout symptomatology and social support at work independent of the private sphere: A population-based study of French teachers. *International Archives of Occupational and Environmental Health*, *92*(6), 891–900. https://doi.org/10.1007/s00420-019-01431-6

Terada, Y. (2023, August 16). *What school leaders can do to support teacher well-being*. Edutopia. https://www.edutopia.org/article/leaders-teacher-wellbeing-action/

The Core Collaborative. (2025). *Sanford B. Dole Middle School: Improving learning in three core subjects*. https://tinyurl.com/2s87zfuz

Thomson, A. L., & Siegel, J. T. (2017). Elevation: A review of scholarship on a moral and other-praising emotion. *The Journal of Positive Psychology*, *12*(6), 628–638. https://doi.org/10.1080/17439760.2016.1269184

Thornton, K. (2025). Embedding a culture of mentoring in a school: A case study. *Journal of Educational Leadership, Policy and Practice*, *39*(1), 1–20. https://doi.org/10.2478/jelpp-2025-0001

Times Educational Supplement. (2025, n.d.). *Selly Park Girls' School wins staff wellbeing school of the year*. https://www.tes.com/schools-awards/uk/winners/2025

Timms, C., Graham, D., & Cottrell, D. (2007). 'I just want to teach'. *Journal of Educational Administration*, *45*(5), 569–586. https://doi.org/10.1108/09578230710778204

Tims, M., Bakker, A. B., & Derks, D. (2013). The impact of job crafting on job demands, job resources, and well-being. *Journal of Occupational Health Psychology*, *18*(2), 230–240. https://doi.org/10.1037/a0032141

Toikka, T., & Tarnanen, M. (2024). A shared vision for a school: Developing a learning community. *Educational Research*, *66*(3), 295–311. https://doi.org/10.1080/00131881.2024.2361412

Travers, C. (2017). Current knowledge on the nature, prevalence, sources and potential impact of teacher stress. In T. M. McIntyre, S. E. McIntyre, & D. J. Francis (Eds.), *Educator stress: An occupational health perspective* (pp. 23–54). Springer.

Tsouloupas, C. N., Carson, R. L., Matthews, R., Grawitch, M. J., & Barber, L. K. (2010). Exploring the association between teachers' perceived student misbehaviour and emotional exhaustion: The importance of teacher efficacy beliefs and emotion regulation. *Educational Psychology*, *30*(2), 173–189. https://doi.org/10.1080/01443410903494460

Tsuyuguchi, K. (2023). Analysis of the determinants of teacher well-being: Focusing on the causal effects of trust relationships. *Teaching and Teacher Education*, *132*, 104240. https://doi.org/10.1016/j.tate.2023.104240

Türktorun, Y. Z., Weiher, G. M., & Horz, H. (2020). Psychological detachment and work-related rumination in teachers: A systematic review. *Educational Research Review*, *31*, 100354. https://doi.org/10.1016/j.edurev.2020.100354

Turner, K., Thielking, M., & Prochazka, N. (2022). Teacher wellbeing and social support: A phenomenological study. *Educational Research*, *64*(1), 77–94. https://doi.org/10.1080/00131881.2021.2013126

Tutar, H., Altınöz, M., & Çakıroğlu, D. (2011). The effects of employee empowerment on achievement motivation and the contextual performance of employees. *African Journal of Business Management*, *5*(15), 6318–6329. https://doi.org/10.5897/AJBM11.085

Tuxford, L. M., & Bradley, G. L. (2014). Emotional job demands and emotional exhaustion in teachers. *Educational Psychology*, *35*(8), 1006–1024. https://doi.org/10.1080/01443410.2014.912260

Ulusoy, N., Mölders, C., Fischer, S., Bayur, H., Deveci, S., Demiral, Y., & Rössler, W. (2016). A matter of psychological safety: Commitment and mental health in Turkish immigrant employees in Germany. *Journal of Cross-Cultural Psychology*, *47*(4), 626–645. https://doi.org/10.1177/0022022115626513

Undie, J., & Nike, A. J. (2016). Teachers class size, job satisfaction and morale in Cross River State secondary schools, Nigeria. *Annals of Modern Education*, *8*(1), 16–26. https://www.ajol.info/index.php/ame/article/view/129651

UNESCO, & International Task Force on Teachers for Education 2030. (2024). *Global report on teachers: Addressing teacher shortages and transforming the profession*. UNESCO. https://doi.org/10.18356/9789231006555

UNESCO. (2023). *Bangladesh institutionalizes the celebration of World Teachers' Day with a vision for educational excellence*. https://tinyurl.com/4erpdrhk

United Nations. (2015). *Transforming our world: The 2030 agenda for sustainable development*. https://sustainabledevelopment.un.org/post2015/transformingourworld/publication

van Dam, A., Noordzij, G., & Born, M. P. (2020). Linking the fit between achievement goal orientation and learning opportunities with employee well-being and absenteeism. *Journal of Personnel Psychology*, *19*(4), 184–196. https://doi.org/10.1027/1866-5888/a000260

van den Heuvel, M., Demerouti, E., & Peeters, M. C. W. (2015). The job crafting intervention: Effects on job resources, self-efficacy, and affective well-being. *Journal of Occupational and Organizational Psychology*, *88*(3), 511–532. https://doi.org/10.1111/joop.12128

Van Maele, D., & Van Houtte, M. (2015). Trust in school: A pathway to inhibit teacher burnout? *Journal of Educational Administration*, *53*(1), 93–115. https://doi.org/10.1108/jea-02-2014-0018

Van Tongeren, D. R., Hibbard, R., Edwards, M., Johnson, E., Diepholz, K., Newbound, H., Shay, A., Houpt, R., Cairo, A., & Green, J. D. (2018). Heroic helping: The effects of priming superhero images on prosociality. *Frontiers in Psychology*, *9*. https://doi.org/10.3389/fpsyg.2018.02243

van Wingerden, J., Bakker, A. B., & Derks, D. (2016). The longitudinal impact of a job crafting intervention. *European Journal of Work and Organizational Psychology*, *26*(1), 107–119. https://doi.org/10.1080/1359432x.2016.1224233

Venema-Steen, I., Southall, A., & Bortoli, A. (2023). Drawing on the locus of control framework to explore the role of school leaders in teacher well-being. *Journal of Educational Research and Practice*, *13*(1). https://doi.org/10.5590/jerap.2023.13.1.11

Vettori, G., Bigozzi, L., Vezzani, C., & Pinto, G. (2022). The mediating role of emotions in the relation between beliefs and teachers' job satisfaction. *Acta Psychologica*, *226*, 103580. https://doi.org/10.1016/j.actpsy.2022.103580

Viac, C., & Fraser, P. (2020, January 1). *Teachers' well-being: A framework for data collection and analysis for PISA and TALIS*. Organisation for Economic Co-operation and Development. http://dx.doi.org/10.1787/c36fc9d3-en

Vianello, M., Galliani, E. M., & Haidt, J. (2010). Elevation at work: The effects of leaders' moral excellence. *The Journal of Positive Psychology*, *5*(5), 390–411. https://doi.org/10.1080/17439760.2010.516764

Vicuña Delos Reyes, J. (2024). Fostering teacher welfare and well-being: Evaluating the school's continuous professional development program. *International Journal of Research Publications*, *152*(1), 171–200. https://doi.org/10.47119/ijrp1001521720246896

Vincent-Höper, S., Teetzen, F., Gregersen, S., & Nienhaus, A. (2017). Leadership and employee well-being. In R. J. Burke & K. M. Page (Eds.), *Research handbook on work and well-being* (pp. 269–291). Edward Elgar Publishing. https://doi.org/10.4337/9781785363269.00021

Vogt, K., Hakanen, J. J., Brauchli, R., Jenny, G. J., & Bauer, G. F. (2015). The consequences of job crafting: A three-wave study. *European Journal of Work and Organizational Psychology*, *25*(3), 353–362. https://doi.org/10.1080/1359432x.2015.1072170

Wagner, L., Baumann, N., & Hank, P. (2015). Enjoying influence on others: Congruently high implicit and explicit power motives are related to teachers' well-being. *Motivation and Emotion*, *40*(1), 69–81. https://doi.org/10.1007/s11031-015-9516-8

Walker, T. D. (2014, June 30). *How Finland keeps kids focused through free play*. The Atlantic. https://www.theatlantic.com/education/archive/2014/06/how-finland-keeps-kids-focused/373544/

Walter, H. L., Kutscher, E. L., Fox, H. B., Tuckwiller, E. D., & Ball, K. B. (2023). A tale of caution: Navigating special education teacher resistance to well-being professional development. *International Journal of Educational Research Open*, *4*, 100253. https://doi.org/10.1016/j.ijedro.2023.100253

Wang, X., & Chen, Z. (2022). 'It hits the spot': The impact of a professional development program on English teacher wellbeing in underdeveloped regions. *Frontiers in Psychology*, *13*. https://doi.org/10.3389/fpsyg.2022.848322

Wang, H., Hall, N. C., & King, R. B. (2021). A longitudinal investigation of teachers' emotional labor, well-being, and perceived student engagement. *Educational Psychology*, *41*(10), 1319–1336. https://doi.org/10.1080/01443410.2021.1988060

Wang, H., Hall, N. C., Goetz, T., & Frenzel, A. C. (2016). Teachers' goal orientations: Effects on classroom goal structures and emotions. *British Journal of Educational Psychology*, *87*(1), 90–107. https://doi.org/10.1111/bjep.12137

Waters, L. (2012). Predicting job satisfaction: Contributions of individual gratitude and institutionalized gratitude. *Psychology*, *3*, 1174–1176. https://doi.org/10.4236/psych.2012.312A173

Watkins, T., Kleshinski, C., Longmire, N., & He, W. (2022). How and when employees proactively extend the benefits of past positive work events to coworkers. *Academy of Management Proceedings*, *2022*(1). https://doi.org/10.5465/ambpp.2022.10484abstract

Watson, A. (2017a, February 12). *From burnout to teacher of the year: Pam's story of loving her job again*. Truth for Teachers. https://truthforteachers.com/truth-for-teachers-podcast/from-burnout-to-teacher-of-the-year/

Watson, A. (2017b, August 13). *Your classroom does not have to be Pinterest-worthy: Stay reflective on the why & avoid comparison.* Truth for Teachers. https://truthforteachers.com/truth-for-teachers-podcast/avoid-comparison/?utm_source=chatgpt.com

Watt, H. M. G., & Richardson, P. W. (2020). Motivation of higher education faculty: (How) it matters! *International Journal of Educational Research*, *100*, 101533. https://doi.org/10.1016/j.ijer.2020.101533

Weigelt, O., Schmitt, A., Syrek, C. J., & Ohly, S. (2021). Exploring the engaged worker over time: A week-level study of how positive and negative work events affect work engagement. *International Journal of Environmental Research and Public Health*, *18*(13), 6699. https://doi.org/10.3390/ijerph18136699

Weiland, A. (2021). Teacher well-being: Voices in the field. *Teaching and Teacher Education*, *99*, 103250. https://doi.org/10.1016/j.tate.2020.103250

Wendsche, J., Ghadiri, A., Bengsch, A., & Wegge, J. (2017). Antecedents and outcomes of nurses' rest break organization: A scoping review. *International Journal of Nursing Studies*, *75*, 65–80. https://doi.org/10.1016/j.ijnurstu.2017.07.005

Wendsche, J., Lohmann-Haislah, A., & Wegge, J. (2016). The impact of supplementary short rest breaks on task performance: A meta-analysis. *Sozialpolitik.ch*, 2, 1–24. https://doi.org/10.18753/2297-8224-75

Wendsche, J., Varol, Y. Z., & Ullmann, S. (2023). Schulpausen: Wie Grundschullehrkräfte in der Ruhe Kraft finden können [School breaks: How primary school teachers can find strength in quiet]. *Grundschule aktuell*, *163*, 29–33.

Wepfer, A. G., Allen, T. D., Brauchli, R., Jenny, G. J., & Bauer, G. F. (2017). Work–life boundaries and well-being: Does work-to-life integration impair well-being through lack of recovery? *Journal of Business and Psychology*, *33*(6), 727–740. https://doi.org/10.1007/s10869-017-9520-y

Westover, J. H. (2025). Employee recognition: An essential facet of ethical leadership and organizational wellbeing. *Human Capital Leadership Review*, *20*(3). https://doi.org/10.70175/hclreview.2020.20.3.6

Wickström, G., & Bendix, T. (2000). The 'Hawthorne effect': What did the original Hawthorne studies actually show? *Scandinavian Journal of Work, Environment & Health*, 26(4), 363–367. http://www.jstor.org/stable/40967074

Wightwick, A. (2022, June 22). *What teachers in Wales make of the controversial changes set to completely change how and what pupils.* Wales Online. https://www.walesonline.co.uk/news/education/wales-education-news-exams-curriculum-23769446

Wiita, T. (2021, January 29). *South metro teacher turns to chalk to make students' day.* KSTP News. https://kstp.com/kstp-news/local-news/south-metro-teacher-turns-to-chalk-to-make-students39-day/

Wikipedia. (2025). *Ceibal project.* https://en.wikipedia.org/wiki/Ceibal_project

Williams, L. A. (2018). Emotions of excellence: Communal and agentic functions of pride, moral elevation, and admiration. In H. C. Lench (Ed.), *The function of emotions: When and why emotions help us* (pp. 235–252). Springer International Publishing. https://doi.org/10.1007/978-3-319-77619-4_12

Winkler, E., Busch, C., Clasen, J., & Vowinkel, J. (2014). Changes in leadership behaviors predict changes in job satisfaction and well-being in low-skilled workers. *Journal of Leadership & Organizational Studies*, *22*(1), 72–87. https://doi.org/10.1177/1548051814527771

Winy Nila, W. (2024). Playfulness and teacher's selfefficacy of early childhood teachers. *Journal of Southeast Asia Psychology*, *12*(1), 15. https://doi.org/10.51200/sapj.v12i1.5053

Wood, P., & Quickfall, A. (2024). Was 2021–2022 an annus horribilis for teacher educators? Reflections on a survey of teacher educators. *British Educational Research Journal*, *50*(5), 2172–2197. https://doi.org/10.1002/berj.4017

World Bank Group. (2023). *Ceibal: Increasing access to digital technology and ensuring education for all in Uruguay.* Transformational Technologies for Human Capital. https://tinyurl.com/yd5aysz6

Wößmann, L. (2007). International evidence on school competition, autonomy, and accountability: A review. *Peabody Journal of Education*, *82*(2–3), 473–497. https://doi.org/10.1080/01619560701313176

Wu, Y., Lai, S. L., & He, S. (2022). Psychological capital of teachers of English as a foreign language and classroom management: Well-being as a mediator. *Social Behavior and Personality: An international Journal*, *50*(12), 1–9. https://doi.org/10.2224/sbp.11916

Xu, Y., & Wang, J. (2024). The mediating role of teaching enthusiasm in the relationship between mindfulness, growth mindset, and psychological well-being of Chinese EFL teachers. *Humanities and Social Sciences Communications*, *11*(1), 1176. https://doi.org/10.1057/s41599-024-03694-y

Yang, H., Liang, C., Liang, Y., Yang, Y., Chi, P., Zeng, X., & Wu, Q. (2023). Association of gratitude with individual and organizational outcomes among volunteers: An application of broaden-and-build theory of positive emotions. *Sage Open*, *13*(4), 21582440231210372. https://doi.org/10.1177/21582440231210372

Yang, N. (2022). An investigation into the interplay between Chinese EFL teachers' emotional intelligence, ambiguity tolerance, and work engagement *Frontiers in Psychology*, *13*. https://doi.org/10.3389/fpsyg.2022.929933

Yin, H., Huang, S., & Lv, L. (2018). A multilevel analysis of job characteristics, emotion regulation, and teacher well-being: A job demands–resources model. *Frontiers in Psychology*, *9*. https://doi.org/10.3389/fpsyg.2018.02395

Yin, H., Huang, S., & Wang, W. (2016). Work environment characteristics and teacher well-being: The mediation of emotion regulation strategies. *International Journal of Environmental Research and Public Health*, *13*(9), 907. https://doi.org/10.3390/ijerph13090907

Yoon, J. S. (2002). Teacher characteristics as predictors of teacher–student relationships: Stress, negative affect, and self-efficacy. *Social Behavior and Personality: An International Journal*, *30*(5), 485–493. https://doi.org/10.2224/sbp.2002.30.5.485

Yu, X., Lin, X., Xue, D., & Zhou, H. (2024). Impact of work engagement on teachers' workplace well-being: A serial mediation model of perceived organizational support and psychological empowerment. *Sage Open*, *14*(4). https://doi.org/10.1177/21582440241291344

Yu, Y.-J. (2023, September 18). As more schools switch to 4-day weeks, will teachers stay? *ABC News*. https://tinyurl.com/y973tvsf

Yuan, K., Le, V.-N., McCaffrey, D. F., Marsh, J. A., Hamilton, L. S., Stecher, B. M., & Springer, M. G. (2013). Incentive pay programs do not affect teacher motivation or reported practices. *Educational Evaluation and Policy Analysis*, *35*(1), 3–22. https://doi.org/10.3102/0162373712462625

Yurt, E. (2022). Collective teacher self-efficacy and burnout: The mediator role of job satisfaction. *International Journal of Modern Education Studies*, *6*(1), 51–69. https://doi.org/10.51383/ijonmes.2022.168

Zarate, K., Maggin, D. M., & Passmore, A. (2019). Meta-analysis of mindfulness training on teacher well-being. *Psychology in the Schools*, *56*(10), 1700–1715. https://doi.org/10.1002/pits.22308

Zarrinabadi, N., Jamalvandi, B., & Rezazadeh, M. (2023). Investigating fixed and growth teaching mindsets and self-efficacy as predictors of language teachers' burnout and professional identity. *Language Teaching Research*, 0(0). 1–19. https://doi.org/10.1177/13621688231151787

Zausmer, T., Dahan, O., & Sasson, I. (2024). Exploring the relationship between teachers' flow-state and learning spaces: Unraveling the impact of design conditions. *Cogent Education*, *11*(1), 2424155. https://doi.org/10.1080/2331186X.2024.2424155

Zee, M., & Koomen, H. M. Y. (2016). Teacher self-efficacy and its effects on classroom processes, student academic adjustment, and teacher well-being. *Review of Educational Research*, *86*(4), 981–1015. https://doi.org/10.3102/0034654315626801

Zeng, G., Chen, X., Cheung, H. Y., & Peng, K. (2019). Teachers' growth mindset and work engagement in the Chinese educational context: Well-being and perseverance of effort as mediators. *Frontiers in Psychology*, *10*. https://doi.org/10.3389/fpsyg.2019.00839

Zerna, C. A. (2025). Teachers' point of views on the implementation of DO No.5, S.2024: Basis for policy review. *Psychology and Education: A Multidisciplinary Journal*, *41*, 713–722. https://doi.org/10.70838/pemj.410604

Zhaleh, K., Ghonsooly, B., & Pishghadam, R. (2018). Effects of conceptions of intelligence and ambiguity tolerance on teacher burnout: A case of Iranian EFL teachers. *Journal of Research in Applied Linguistics*, *9*, 118–140. https://doi.org/10.22055/rals.2018.13796

Zheng, X., Huang, H., & Yu, Q. (2024). The associations among gratitude, job crafting, teacher–student relationships, and teacher psychological well-being. *Frontiers in Psychology*, *15*. https://doi.org/10.3389/fpsyg.2024.1329782

Zhou, S., Slemp, G. R., & Vella-Brodrick, D. A. (2024). Factors associated with teacher wellbeing: A meta-analysis. *Educational Psychology Review*, *36*(2). https://doi.org/10.1007/s10648-024-09886-x

Zilka, A., Nussbaum, S., & Bogler, R. (2023). The relationships among growth mindset, flow, critically reflective behavior and teacher burnout. *International Journal of School & Educational Psychology*, *11*(4), 367–379. https://doi.org/10.1080/21683603.2023.2245372

Zinsser, K. M., Christensen, C. G., & Torres, L. (2016). She's supporting them; who's supporting her? Preschool center-level social–emotional supports and teacher well-being. *Journal of School Psychology*, *59*, 55–66. https://doi.org/10.1016/j.jsp.2016.09.001

www.ingramcontent.com/pod-product-compliance
Lightning Source LLC
LaVergne TN
LVHW010615100826
845148LV00014B/2985

* 9 7 8 1 8 3 7 4 2 0 6 0 5 *